BODY WEIGHT BASICS

A Beginner's Guide To Resistance Training

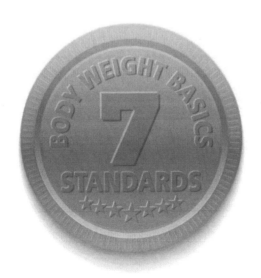

ROSS CLIFFORD & ASHLEY KALYM

First published in 2019
Kindle Direct Publishing

Photographs Matt Marsh
Text Design Ashley Kalym
Cover Design Ashley Kalym
ISBN 9781093567236

CONTENTS

Performing the Triceps Dip
Ledge Dip with Bent Legs
Ledge Dip With Straight Legs
Kneeling Triceps Push-up
Shallow Triceps Dip
Negative Triceps Dip
Assisted Triceps Dip

10.4 Standard Four: The Squat

The Anatomy Of The Squat
Key Features Of The Squat
Performing the Squat
Sit Stand
Shallow Squat
Shallow One Legged Squat
Crouch
Assisted Squat
Deep Squat Position

10.5 Standard Five: The Lunge

The Anatomy Of The Lunge
Key Features Of The Lunge
Performing the Lunge
Step Stand
Hip Flexor Stretch
Lateral Lunge
Shallow Lunge
Lunge Balance
Static Lunge

10.6 Standard Six: The Plank

The Anatomy Of The Plank
Key Features Of The Plank
Performing the Plank
Prone Pelvic Tilt
Platform Push-up Hold
Bridge
Kneeling Plank
Static Crunch
Plank Pulses

1. Preface

'What if someone is unable to do the most basic of body weight exercises before attempting to move on to more complex or tougher exercises?'

This was the question we puzzled over before further asking, 'everyone can do a push-up, can't they?' But then we wondered about how well someone could perform a push-up and we both thought about our experiences in physiotherapy and personal training. We concluded that not everyone can do a proper push-up, but they may be able to do ten or even twenty dubious push-ups. We thought about the consequences of this in terms of injury potential and the inability to progress to more complex body weight exercises. It was obvious that being able to complete ten dubious push-ups would be a self-limiting and possibly detrimental process. Then we got started on the pull-up. That's when we realised there was a need to educate and inform on the techniques that are the bedrock of good quality body weight exercise. That was the moment we conceived the concept of this book – Body Weight Basics.

So we had the push-up and pull-up in the bag; two obvious candidates for a book about mastering the physical attributes for foundational exercise. But what about the rest? What else should we include and when should we stop? We sat down and began to list what we thought would be an endless programme of basic body weight exercises. We got as far as seven! But we really wanted eight (because we liked the idea of an 'Essential Eight'). When we tried to add more we asked ourselves, 'what does this exercise add that someone short on time, energy or motivation couldn't get from the others in order to progress to more difficult exercises?' We pondered the seven for a while. It didn't seem such a bad number. There were Seven Wonders of the World, the Magnificent Seven, and then there was Snow White... OK, perhaps the last example was not the most convincing. But seven seemed right. It was the days of the week and the colours of the rainbow. And so the 'Seven Standards' of body weight exercise was born.

Once we had our Seven Standards we set about planning the exercises that would be complementary to achieving our benchmarks. We used objects around the house to test the difficulty and accessibility of these 'preparatory' exercises, as they became known. We played around with variations of push-ups on a kitchen floor, tested triceps dips on the seats and backs of dining chairs, and practiced pull-ups on the frame of a children's swing. It was definitely accessible, it was achievable in stages, and it was great fun. We also discovered we both needed to work on our low-back and hamstring flexibility when we got round to the Downward Dog. As we wrote down our preparatory exercises for each Standard an obvious pattern emerged. We seemed naturally to come to rest after a total of seven exercises within each Standard. And so once again the world's favourite number seemed to work its magic, and like J. K. Rowling and her Harry Potter books, we stopped at seven.

We hope you find this book useful and that you enjoy practicing the exercises as much as we enjoyed putting them together. Towards the end of the book you will find training programs that cover the Seven Standards and provide well-rounded exercise routines. The programs are also graded to give you a sense of achievement and progression, so that when you can complete the Seven Standards of Body Weight Basics you will know you have done something worthwhile.

Master the basics, and who knows where that will take you!

Ross and Ashley.

2. The Goal Of This Book

The goal of Body Weight Basics is to teach you how to get stronger and progress your physical capabilities. Measuring these results is very important, and as such you will need to have goals to aim for. There are some body weight exercises that can be thought of as "standards": those movements that should be in the repertoire of every person that exercises their body. Although there are hundreds, if not thousands of body weight exercises, there are only a handful that can be thought of as providing an essential standard of fitness.

With our combined knowledge and experience in physical training and rehabilitation we found that the following exercises would be enough to provide well-rounded strength, stability and range of motion around joints. These exercises are the push-up, the pull-up, the triceps dip, the squat, the lunge, the plank, and the inverted shoulder press. These seven exercises collectively use most of the muscles of the body to create a balanced physique that will provide a solid foundation for most physical tasks. We have come to the call them the "Seven Standards" of body weight exercise. They are the bedrock of Body Weight Basics.

Each section of this book related to the Seven Standards takes the same format to improve usability and familiarity. It starts with a justification of the Standard, followed by some basic anatomy to give context to the exercise. After that we get down to business; a full description of the each of the "Standards", complete with photographic illustration and teaching points. Each of the Seven Standards forms part of a series of seven exercises developed to maximise your achievement. These 'Preparatory' exercises are clearly explained and are demonstrated in high quality photographs.

We have endeavoured to make learning the movements as easy as possible, with advice on how to progress in line with your own abilities. Even if you are a complete beginner who has never trained before, with little to no strength, you will be able to perform the first Preparatory exercise that accompanies each Standard, and from there progress steadily towards achievement of the Standards as your body grows stronger and more physically capable.

3. Why Body Weight Exercise?

You may be thinking about why we have chosen body weight exercise, and not free-weight exercise, or exercise using machines, or aerobics, or any other of the hundreds of different types of physical training. Throughout this book we will justify the selected exercises and we will also explain why body weight exercise is a great form of training for novices and those more familiar with exercise training.

Personal Experience

We are both huge fans of body weight exercise, and have benefited greatly from performing it. We have seen first hand how it has helped our physical performance, both in sport and in our daily lives. We have used it to restore function after injury and to 'bulletproof' ourselves against future injury.

Ashley has also written an entire book dedicated to body weight training, with a huge range of exercises moving from the very easy to the very hard. *Complete Calisthenics - The Ultimate Guide To Bodyweight Exercise*, is a book that you can graduate to after mastering the Standards set out in *Body Weight Basics*.

Highly Accessible

Body weight training is highly accessible and adaptable, making it suitable for all ages and abilities. Absolute beginners can perform many of the movements in the arena of body weight exercise, even if it is in a simplified format. Other body weight movements require so much strength that only a select few have the ability to perform them. That is the spectrum of this method of training; from *Body Weight Basics* to *Complete Calisthenics*.

Minimal Equipment

As body weight exercise requires little if any equipment, it can be performed at home or when traveling. Body weight exercise is cost and time effective, saving you money on gym memberships, and working multiple muscles at any one time to maximise your workout. If the atmosphere of a gym is something that makes you feel uncomfortable then being able to work out from home means that you will always be comfortable exercising. You'll be the judge of your efforts and results.

Of course, there are some exercises that require additional equipment (the pull-up, for example). This is normally where the exercise requires a solid base for the body to move against, and this may need to be at a certain height or of a particular size and shape. Pushing, squatting, jumping, and core type exercises more often than not require no equipment at all.

Transferable Fitness

Although the term functional fitness has seen huge popularity over the last decade or so, the label can definitely be attached to body weight exercise. If you are wondering what functional fitness means, it is simply the usefulness that an exercise imparts in everyday life. For example, the ability to do a body weight squat is extremely useful in many everyday situations. Sitting down and standing up, climbing stairs, picking objects up and chasing after your children are all tasks that are made easier by the fact that you can squat properly. Body weight exercise is perhaps the best example of transferable strength-based fitness, and therefore functional fitness, and may help you in many ways in your everyday activities.

Building Strength

Although cardiovascular exercise gets most of the media attention when it comes to bettering health and improving function in life, many incredible benefits can be found with strength training. Strength training does what you think it might do; makes you stronger. But what is strength?

Strength is the ability of muscles to *exert* force. If you want to lift something, push something, or physically interact with the world around you then you will need strength. Your life habits and needs will dictate how much strength is adequate for you individually, but in very few instances is it beneficial to be weaker. Overall, it is better to be stronger, and the various forms of strength training can help you to achieve this.

You will see throughout this book that there are many advantages to developing or maintaining muscle strength, from preventing age-related muscle loss to improving posture. You may be an older adult seeking to reduce your risk of falls, or a young adult wanting to develop the aesthetics of your physique. Pushing and pulling against the resistance created by your own body weight will contribute greatly to all of these goals!

Another definition of strength is the ability to *withstand* force. The authors have addressed this extensively elsewhere (*Bulletproof Bodies: Body weight Exercise for Injury Prevention and Rehabilitation*), but in short if you are better able to withstand the effects of external and internal forces on body structures then you are less likely to be injured or suffer aches and pains.

Why Not Cardiovascular?

In the previous section we espoused the benefits of strength training over cardiovascular training, but this does not mean that 'cardio' is not beneficial. In fact we actively encourage you to take regular cardiovascular physical activity or exercise to supplement your strength training, but such a topic is just not within the scope of this book.

Improving the strength and efficiency of the heart and lungs is beneficial to many aspects of health. Current government recommendations in the UK are for adults to undertake 150 minutes of moderate physical activity or 75 minutes of vigorous activity per week, or a combination of the two. This should be in bouts of no less than 10 minutes. And guess what? - strength training should be included *at least* twice a week! You've got that one covered if you apply the principles of this book.

4. Exercise Terminology

Being new to exercise can be daunting, especially with all of the new terminology that you may come across. However, the number of terms that you need to understand is quite small, and the terms themselves can be fairly self-explanatory. To help you we have included an explanation of the most common words and phrases that you need to know.

Range Of Motion

All exercises that require your joints to move have a range of motion, or ROM for short. Range of motion refers to how far your joints move when performing a movement or exercise. If we take the push-up as an example, a *small range of motion* would be if your elbows reached 90 degrees of bend. A *large range of motion* would be if your chest touched the ground. In general, a smaller range of motion is easier, and a larger range of motion is harder. This is very useful to know as adjusting the range of motion can be used to make exercises suitable for a wide range of abilities.

Reps

Rep is short for 'repetition' and means the number of times that you do an exercise consecutively before taking a rest. For example, 'squat for 10 reps' means to perform 10 squats in a row without stopping.

Sometimes you may see exercises that are not performed for reps, but instead are held for a certain length of time. An example of this is the plank (Standard Six). You might hold the plank for 30 seconds before resting, instead of doing a certain number of reps.

Sets

'Sets' means the number of times you do a group of reps (repetitions). For example, you may see '3 sets of 10 reps'. This means that you would do 10 reps of an exercise (the first set) before resting, then do another 10 reps (the second set) before resting again. Finally you would do another 10 reps (the third set) before resting. Each set is normally followed by a rest period to allow the muscles or the cardiovascular system to recover slightly before starting the following set.

Sets and reps will almost always be written together, and you will see instructions like, *'3 sets of 5 reps'*, or *'10 sets of 10 reps'* and so on. These instructions may also be written as *1 x 20*, or *3 x 15*, or *5 x 5*, where the first value is the number of sets, and the second value is the number of reps in each set.

Hold Times

Certain exercises (like the plank - Standard Six) are not performed for reps, as they do not have any movement. In these types of exercises a set time period is used instead of a number of reps. For example, a plank performed for 3 sets of 30 seconds would go as follows: hold the plank for 30 seconds, then rest, then hold for another 30 seconds, then rest again, and then hold for the final set of 30 seconds.

Rest Time

In the exercise programs offered in this book you will see a value referred to as 'rest time'. Rest time is the time taken between each set, in order to allow your muscles to recover enough for the next set, or the next exercise. Rest time is typically between 30 to 90 seconds for strength training, depending on the exercise that you are performing. Strength exercises that are a little easier, or which put less stress on the muscles will require less rest time, and those exercises that put more of a demand on the body will require more. A high intensity of work will also require a longer rest time, as will some forms of cardiovascular exercise.

It is important to know that the rest times that we list are adjustable, depending on your ability and fitness level. For example, for the push-up group of exercises we recommend 30 to 60 seconds rest between each set, but if you are a complete beginner, you may need 90 to 120 seconds to fully recover before the next set. If you are progressing well, and feel you don't need the full 30 seconds of rest, then take less. Just be sure that you have recovered sufficiently to get full effort in the following set.

5. Principles Of Exercise

When beginning exercise it is beneficial to understand some fundamental principles of training, so that you better understand how and why your exercise routine is structured the way it is. This way you will appreciate why the suggested numbers of sets and reps is making you stronger.

Resistance

The dictionary definition of 'resistance' is: the stopping effect exerted by one material thing on another. Sounds complicated, right? When talking about exercise, 'resistance' is simply the force felt when pushing, pulling, lifting, or working against a weight or gravity. In other words, it is the opposing force that wants to stop your joints moving through their range. When you push open a heavy door the door is resisting your efforts to push it open. When you lift something off the ground the force of gravity acting on the mass of the object is resisting your attempt to lift the object.

When working with body weight exercise, gravity and your own body mass combine to form the resistance you feel. In Body Weight Basics we show you how you can manipulate your body weight by adjusting joint angles and body position. If we take the push-up as our example, then you will feel resistance in a number of different ways. You will feel resistance in your hands as gravity pulls on the mass of your upper body. You will feel resistance around your waist and in your core muscles as gravity tries to pull your hips to the ground. And that's just the start position! Once you start moving you will feel resistance in the muscles of your upper body as they work to push you back up to the start position. If it turns out that your mass plus gravity creates too much resistance we will show you how to adjust those joint angles and body positions to help you achieve your goals.

Progressive Overload

Now that you know what resistance is, and why your muscles, tendons and joints adapt to the resistance created by your body weight, we need to consider how these adaptations become progressive.

'Progressive' in this context means to increase or advance. *Progressive overload* is when you gradually increase the amount of resistance that your body is subjected to in order to continually increase the gains in performance. These gains could be muscle strength, muscle endurance, balance, speed, power, flexibility, joint ROM, or even cardiovascular endurance. Over an extended amount of time (weeks, months, and even years), you would need to

14

progressively increase the workout load by increasing the resistance, ROM or distance travelled, for example.

With regard to body weight training your body will continue to get stronger as long as the amount of resistance it works against also increases over time. In Body Weight Basics there are six preparatory exercises behind each of the Seven Standards of body weight exercise. These preparatory exercises and their Standard have varying requirements for strength, balance and joint ROM. Towards the end of this book we have generated several training programs that can be used sequentially to create progressive overload. Remember to progress at your own pace and enjoy the gains along the way!

Regression

Regression is simply a technical way of saying 'to move backwards'. For the effects of exercise to last then you must continue to exercise, and to exercise close to the levels of that which you have previously done. As the saying goes; 'if you don't use it, you lose it'. The human body is a relatively energy efficient and 'lean' machine. All of its processes compete for the nutrients taken in daily, from the beating of the heart and conduction of nerve impulses, to the contraction of muscles.

Growth takes a large proportion of this energy intake, and this includes the growth of skeletal muscle (see the following section on Hypertrophy). But consider this - if you don't need larger and stronger muscles anymore in order to cope with a resistance training programme you have abandoned then why would the body continue to support their growth? The answer is that it won't continue to fuel the growth of these muscles. It will break them down and recycle their building blocks (you may have heard of amino acids!), and so your muscle mass will regress, and so too will your physical capabilities. If you don't want to lose it, use it!

Overtraining

As important as exercise is, there is always the risk that overtraining can occur. Overtraining involves training so much that damage is done to the body without adequate time or energy available for recovery. When the stress on the body from exercise exceeds the ability to recover then training gains become less. There may be a plateau or even a decrease in physical performance. Imagine that; training much harder than ever and getting worse! Who would do such a thing?

Unfortunately many people move unknowingly into overtraining territory. Some of this may be a lack of knowledge, some perhaps related to other life events like work or diet that are unable to support a busy training schedule. On a more serious note some causes of overtraining include exercise addiction. People can become addicted to exercise, whether this is psychological fixation with some aspect of exercising or whether it is the internal body chemistry responding to the molecular effects of exercise. If at any time you think you may fall into this category of overtraining then we suggest you seek assessment from a suitably qualified health or medical professional.

In addition to the more serious forms of overtraining there is also the type caused by a monotonous training programme. When the body is doing the same exercise routine over and over again the nervous system accommodates to the regular stress, and the lack of training stimulus leads to less gains and a feeling of apathy towards training. In such instances we recommend mixing up your training schedule regularly, and to help with this we have provided a variety of training programs at the back of this book.

Keep an eye out for overtraining by monitoring your body and training results for the following:

• Irritability
• Low mood
• The feeling of 'Burnout'
• Persistent fatigue.
• Persistent muscle soreness
• Raised heart rate at rest
• Increased occurrence in infections like coughs, colds and sore throats
• Increased incidence of injuries
• Reduced physical performance
• Prolonged recovery
• Unable to complete workouts

If you suspect that you are heading towards overtraining then check your diet for the right quantity and quality of food. Are you getting sufficient calories and consuming a diet with the proteins, vitamins and minerals needed for repair and growth? Consider also taking a break from your training program or reduce the intensity or volume of your training. Keep a diary of your training plans and look back over large periods of the year - could you vary the training over periods related to other life events. Check your sleep quality and quantity. We offer further advice on this elsewhere in the book.

Ultimately you are training to improve yourself in some way. You should never become a slave to your training program and if you begin to lose interest or motivation, or notice you are failing to progress then come back to this section of the book and then take a look at your relationship with exercise.

Frequency

Like you, both authors lead busy lives and so we fully understand how difficult it can be to make time to exercise. People can convince themselves that the time to exercise just does not exist in their schedules. They have children, a demanding job, friends they need to keep in contact with, and wider family demands. All these things genuinely require their attention. We are realistic people and we totally understand that few people have surplus hours to devote to exercise. But, don't you owe it to yourself, your children, your wider family, your friends (and possibly even your employer) to take care of yourself and keep yourself well? Who will do all of the above when you are burned-out and susceptible to physical and psychological ill-health?

This is where Body Weight Basics comes to your rescue. The exercises in this book that have become our Seven Standards take little time to perform, and in just three sessions per week you will begin to see real benefits. Completing approximately 30 minutes per session of Body Weight Basics programmes means that in 1 ½ hours a week you will get the fitness benefits you deserve. That's 90 minutes out of your entire week! Of course, if you want more benefits you will need to put in more time but we suggest a maximum of three hours per week would bring huge gains.

No matter how busy your life, dedicating 90 to 180 minutes a week to improving your physical strength and resilience is justifiable. Devoting this amount of time to exercise is achievable if you prioritise it.

If you really are tight for time, try thinking about things you can cut out of your daily routine that you see little to no benefit from. Ashley realised that he was spending more time on Instagram than he really needed and that he could free up at least an hour a week by logging off sooner. Ross found that when his children were small he could be creative and use his play time with them as his exercise time - with the children sitting on his back whilst doing push-ups or pressing them above his head. Please consider safety if doing the latter!

Listening To Your Body

One of the most useful skills that you can develop when starting to exercise is to learn to listen to your body. Listening to your body means to know when to push hard, when to go easy, and when to rest. This skill is not learned overnight; rather it is learned with experience, and the longer you exercise, the better you will get at listening to your body. As you progress, this skill will become increasingly valuable, especially if you move on from the exercises in this book to more advanced movements (see *Complete Calisthenics* by Ashley).

You will benefit by learning to listen to your body when you are exercising. This is important because you need to learn to tell how hard you are working, in order to be able to apply the correct amount of effort. For example, let's say you are doing pull-ups. This is a tough exercise and requires great effort and strain, but does it require 80% of your maximum effort? 90%? 100%? Being able to judge how much more you have left in the tank is vital in being able to know your limits, and to be able to reach above them. One way of developing this is to place enough strain on your body that you are only able to complete one repetition of the exercise. This will give you a feel for 100% effort. You can also consider the level of 'perceived' exertion. When completing any exercise compare how you think it feels with an exercise that was "flat out". The easiest method to quantify this is to think of a rating scale of 1 to 10, where 10 is maximum effort. Valid and reliable scales exist for this but a review of these is beyond the scope of this book.

6. Responses To Exercise

If you are new to exercise, or have limited experience with physical activity, then some of your body's responses may seem alien, or may even have you feeling concerned. In this section we are going to look at the various ways your body responds to exercise, to better understand what you should feel as a normal response to exercise.

DOMS

Delayed onset muscle soreness, or DOMS as we shall refer to it, is an ache felt in muscles after exercise. You may be familiar with this sensation already if you have dabbled in exercise previously. It may even have put you off exercise in the past.

DOMS is experienced after unaccustomed exercise and is usually felt about one to two days after the bout of activity. It is a perfectly normal response to exercise and is even experienced by those who exercise regularly. The key word here is 'unaccustomed' exercise, meaning something not done for a while (or ever) or not done to the current degree of effort. Therefore if you are going at your body weight exercise routine too aggressively then it is more likely you will experience the ache and stiffness in muscles that is DOMS. Even if you've been doing body weight exercise for a while and then one day you decide to vary or progress the intensity of your workout then you may have DOMS in the days that follow.

So, is DOMS something to be worried about? The answer is generally 'no'. It may be uncomfortable but it should not put you off your exercise programme. Although DOMS is the result of low-level muscle trauma following exercise it is actually the stimulus for muscle growth! The body will only repair itself to become stronger if there is a need for it to do so. The muscle strain caused by exercise is the stimulus for the body to get stronger to better deal with that strain (lifting your body weight).

We should point out a few things about DOMS before you embark on your Body Weight Basics programme. Firstly, if you are experiencing DOMS after every workout then you are probably going too hard too soon in each session. This may mean that your recovery between sessions will be insufficient and you'll probably end up regressing in your training goals. All your hard work could be wasted in this case. Secondly, DOMS will normally take 24 to 72 hours to peak — hence the term 'delayed'. If you are experiencing muscle pain during or immediately after exercise then this acute muscle soreness may be a sign of too strenuous exercise. Be careful as this could lead to more severe damage to the muscles or tendons.

Hypertrophy

Any word that begins with the prefix 'hyper' means an increase in something, often above 'normal' levels. For example, the term *hyperglycaemic* means an increase in blood sugar, while *hypertension* is an increase in blood pressure, and *hypermobility* means when joints have excessive range of movement.

Hypertrophy is the term that describes the growth of muscle in response to exercise. The exact mechanism is complex and can be found in full in other books, but in brief, exercise that is intense enough to cause minor damage to muscle fibres will lead to the development of thicker and extra muscle fibres. To maximise this process the body requires proper rest and nutrition. The overall response is that your body adapts to better cope with the exercise stress, making the muscles larger and stronger.

The Role Of Rest

As important as exercise is, for the body to repair itself and for you to get stronger, and fitter, rest is perhaps even more important. This might seem strange; after all if you want to lose weight, get fitter, and become stronger, surely you need to spend every waking moment exercising, right?

Wrong! In reality, a few hours of exercise per week is more than enough to ensure great results. Rest is the time when your body is healing and repairing itself from the minor damage that occurs when you exercise. It is important to know that this 'damage' is relatively minor and is a result of the physical stress being placed upon the body. This stress is what signals your body to make adaptations and improvements, in order to become stronger and fitter.

There are a few things for you to consider in terms of the quality and quantity of your rest:

The first is to develop good sleep hygiene; ensuring you get sufficient "good" sleep. For this you need to practice good sleep habits. Go to bed at a similar time every night, preferably before 10pm, avoid screens and phones at least an hour before bed, and sleep in a darkened room to make sure you are able to properly shut off.

Secondly, try and minimize unnecessary stress in your life. This can be very difficult depending on your own personal circumstances. If you find that you are prone to higher levels of psychological stress and worry try practicing meditation or mindfulness.

Enforce proper breaks in your working day, or time-out for yourself. Take regular, short walks outdoors and surround yourself with nature whenever you can, breathing in fresh air.

There are many other techniques out there to help manage psychological stress and its physical manifestations, but they are beyond the scope of this book. One thing we can assure you of is that there is an overwhelming amount of research evidence that supports the use of exercise in helping to manage stress and anxiety. By practicing the body weight exercises in this book you are already on your road to a more restful existence!

7. Eating For Exercise

This section of the book is concerned with diet and nutrition, which is essential for health and for getting the most out of exercise. If you have not exercised much before, then some of the information here may be completely new to you, as will the dietary recommendations.

There are a number of things that will change once you start practicing the exercises in this book. One is your appetite. The amount you feel you need to eat will likely go up, and this is perfectly normal, and in fact, is necessary for your body to repair and grow. A good analogy can be found with your car. If you drive faster your car will require more fuel. If it doesn't receive enough fuel, the engine cannot work, and your car will come to a stop. The same thing happens with the body. If you are exercising regularly and do not eat enough, or often enough, or the right types of food, then your body will not be able to recover properly from exercise.

Appetite

We're not going to lie; if you begin an exercise program your appetite is likely to increase. But if weight-loss is your ultimate goal with exercise then do not worry. This book is by no means an authority on diet, and if you require further information we direct you to other sources, but here we will offer you some simple advice on eating for exercise.

The amount of food you should be looking to eat will need to match, but not necessarily exceed, what your body needs to recover and grow following exercise. And if your training is to be progressive, with increasing gains in strength or endurance, then your food intake may continue to increase accordingly for a while.

When it comes to choosing the types of food to consume then it is best to avoid processed foods. These foods tend to be dense in calories and the type of nutrients contained within may not be helpful to your exercise needs. Natural foods on the other hand are rarely high in calories and have no hidden extras, and so eating huge quantities will help manage your increased appetite without leading to unwanted weight gain. Junk foods for example tend to be heavy in calories and eating enough to feel full often means consuming a large amount of energy.

The exact amount of food you will need to consume will vary depending on a number of factors, and once again we direct you to more authoritative sources on diet for the exact science. In summary you should consider in the equation your age, height, body composition, muscle mass, training history, and your genetics. Every reader will differ with respect to this list.

One thing we all share is the type of nutrients we require, and once again we find the magic number 7: Protein, carbohydrates, fats, fibre (roughage), vitamins, minerals, and water.

Protein

When you are doing regular exercise training it is important to include protein in every meal. Protein has a high satiety rating, keeping you feeling fuller for longer. Protein is the building material of muscle and connective tissues, such as tendons, and these structures will need the raw materials to adapt to the strains of exercise training. Developing your lean-mass by increasing your muscle composition will raise your resting metabolism meaning that even at rest you will be burning more calories and this will help keep your weight under control.

The protein that you consume in your diet, regardless of the source, is made up of building blocks called amino acids. Once digested, these amino acids are reorganized to build new structures within you. When developing the muscle tissue to improve your strength the general daily recommendation is to consume two grams of dietary protein for every kilogram of body weight.

In terms of your proteins, it is best to get it from animal sources, as these contain all of the essential amino acids that the body needs. Try and get the best quality cuts that you can, and if the animal's welfare is important to you, do as much research into the origin of the product as possible. Organic and ethically farmed produce is becoming easier to find, with many more people aware of the benefits of ethically sourced food.

Carbohydrate

Carbohydrate is an important nutrient that contributes to health and exercise performance. It has a history of bad press with many fad diets recommending a complete removal of 'carbs'. It is more important to understand that the source of the carbohydrates is what should be considered. What follows is a very brief overview.

Carbohydrates can be considered in two camps: starchy and non-starchy. Non-starchy carbohydrates provide the energy we need for exercise but are not packed with many calories per unit of food and do not quickly raise blood sugar levels once consumed. Such foods include leafy vegetables, carrots, cauliflower, green beans, sweet corn, and sweet potatoes. Starchy carbohydrates include bread, pasta, potatoes, and rice. They tend to be stodgy, have a denser calorie content, and can contribute to weight gain if eaten in excess. Starchy carbs also include cakes, donuts, and chocolate. Look for alternatives where possible such as brown rice instead of white rice, or sweet potato instead of a normal spud. Especially ones that are chipped and fried!

Above all try and avoid processed or refined carbohydrates. These foods resemble nothing that is naturally occurring and usually come in an attractive wrapper that children can't resist. You may see these products labelled as 'no added sugar', or 'contains natural sugars'. This is where manufacturers get a little naughty! Sugar is a natural substance, found throughout many natural foods. It is how this sugar is delivered to the body that requires attention. Further discussion on this topic is beyond the scope of this book, but there are plenty of information sources out there for you to learn more.

Fats

Fats have received a bad reputation over the last few decades, in part because of a misunderstanding of what they do in the body, and their importance as a result. It is easy to think of fats as making you 'fat', but this is not strictly true. Any excess calories, regardless of what food source they come from will tend to make you gain weight, but cutting out all fats from your diet can often cause more harm than good. There is also good evidence to show that the consumption of modern fats and margarine type spreads are not good for the body, and as a result we would recommend sticking to natural fats, both for cooking and for eating.

Fats are an essential energy source and are required for the synthesis of hormones in the body, and for the structure and function of the cells in your body. Fats come from many sources, mainly animal products such as meat, eggs, dairy, and from certain vegetables, nuts, and legumes, like avocado, cashews, peanuts, and olive oil. These natural sources are better for you than processed or man-made sources, and eating them will help rather than hinder your weight loss and fitness goals.

Fibre

Fibre, or roughage, has an essential role in health, but not necessarily as a nutrient. It helps to keep the digestive system in good working order by adding bulk to the passage of waste through the digestive tract. Sources of fibre include fruits, vegetables, and pulses.

Getting enough fibre in your diet is easy if you eat even moderately healthily. Every time you eat a piece of fruit or a serving of vegetables you will get fibre.

Top tips for getting fibre into the diet include eating some fruit with breakfast, snacking on dried fruit, and having vegetables with every meal.

Vitamins and Minerals

There are many vitamins and minerals needed in the diet for good health and function. A discussion of these is beyond the scope of this book but we will provide an outline of some of these micronutrients that support exercise training.

Weight bearing exercise, which includes all of the exercises in this book, will help build strong, healthy bones. But this process needs to be supported with an adequate amount of calcium in the diet. Calcium is one of the key minerals that hardens the framework of your skeleton. This nutrient is often linked to a dairy-based diet, but there are many dietary sources of calcium. Examples of calcium sources include:

• Milk
• Kale
• Sardines
• Yogurt
• Broccoli
• Watercress
• Cheese
• Bok Choy

Vitamin D is a nutrient that is linked to calcium. Your body needs Vitamin D to be able to process the calcium mentioned above for healthy bones. Vitamin D is found in a range of foods, and a balanced diet should provide sufficient amounts. The body will also make Vitamin D with exposure to sunlight, and so doing your body weight exercise routine outdoors during the day (where possible) will bring added benefits. However, please do not expose yourself to harmful UV rays. Exercising outdoors for 20 minutes a day (with sunscreen if needed) would be our recommendation.

Another vitamin worth mentioning here is Vitamin C. You may be aware that Vitamin C is good for keeping colds away, but actually this effect lacks any real scientific evidence. What you may be less aware of is the effect of vitamin C on soft tissue healing. In section 6 of Body weight Basics we introduced the concept that strength training actually involves causing a small amount of trauma to soft tissues, that then encourages those tissues to adapt to the strain and become stronger. Vitamin C helps in the building of collagen, a protein vital for repairing connective tissues like ligaments and tendons and the general support structures of the body. It also increases the amount of iron absorbed from food, useful in promoting the oxygen carrying capacity of blood. Finally,

Vitamin C is a known antioxidant, protecting your cells from damaging cellular ageing!
A large number of foods contain Vitamin C, including:

• Broccoli
• Papaya
• Bell peppers
• Brussels sprouts
• Strawberries
• Pineapple
• Oranges
• Kiwi Fruit
• Cauliflower
• Grapefruit
• Tomatoes

Water

You may have heard many times that hydration is essential for proper health, and also for proper exercise performance. It is easy to get dehydrated when exercising, especially if you do not drink enough water in the first place.

Water is important because it is the fluid that helps the body to function, at all levels. Your cells are filled with it and are bathed in it, and use it constantly in their biochemical reactions. Your blood is mostly composed of it and it bolsters your blood pressure, while your musculoskeletal system is cushioned and lubricated by the stuff. Water is therefore essential to the proper functioning of every part of your body.

It is important to realise that drinking fluid is not the same as drinking water! You cannot consume a pint of soft drink, or coffee, or fruit juice, and regard it as being equal to consuming the same volume of water. Obviously there is water in soft drinks, coffee, and fruit juice, but it is not pure water and this can affect the flow of this water into your bloodstream and cells. Some of these drinks choices, like coffee, tea and alcohol, are diuretics. Diuretics are substances that cause you to lose water (by visiting the toilet more often)!

To give you some guidance on how much water to consume daily we have included a table showing how much water you should drink. This is based roughly on your body mass. Note that this is not an exact science, as there are many other factors to consider (muscle mass, height, body type, climate, activity level, and diet), that make it impossible for us to advise you on exactly how much to drink. Use this table as a rough guide and drink more/less as required.

Your Weight (lbs)	Your Weight (kg)	Water Intake (l)
100	45.5	1.5
110	50	1.7
120	54.5	1.8
130	59	2
140	64	2.1
150	68	2.3
160	73	2.4
170	77	2.6
180	82	2.7
190	86	2.9
200	91	3
210	95.5	3.2
220	100	3.3
230	104.5	3.5
240	109	3.6
250	113.5	3.8
260	118	3.9
270	122.5	4.1
280	127	4.2
290	132	4.4
300	136.5	4.5

If you are some way off consuming this daily amount and decide that you need to increase your intake then you must build up gradually. Drinking high volumes of water when your body is not used to it can overload your systems and dilute your cells. This can have very dangerous consequences. If nothing else you will be running to the toilet more often! Build up slowly and consult your doctor if you have concerns.

8. Preparing To Exercise

Starting an exercise routine can be daunting, but by preparing yourself physically and psychology you can reduce some of the concerns. In this section we will discuss some ways in which you can prepare for exercise training.

Understand Your Limitations

Exercising and getting stronger and fitter are all about overcoming real and perceived barriers, some of which may be your current physical limitations. In order to do this it is important to realise what your own physical limitations are before starting an exercise routine.

The different levels of ability that people have are extremely varied, and it is unrealistic to compare yourself to someone else. They may have been training for years, they may have a history of competitive sport, they may have a very different body shape, and perhaps most importantly they will have their own motivations for training. When starting to exercise we would recommend starting small and building up gradually. That way you will always feel like you are progressing and achieving, by comparing yourself with a previous version of yourself.

If you are confident that the first stage of each preparatory exercise will be too easy for you, we suggest you do the stage anyway. The best-case scenario is that you will blast through them and be given a huge confidence boost. The worst-case scenario is that the exercise will surprise you with its difficulty, and you will better understand the level of your abilities.

Moving ahead too fast too soon can potentially cause many problems. If you try a variation that is too advanced first, this can be demotivating, and can also expose the body to forces that it is not ready for, risking injury. If you find yourself battling with injuries that have niggled you in the past then we recommend the book *Bulletproof Bodies - Body Weight Exercise For Injury Prevention And Rehabilitation*, written specifically by the authors to address injury resistance and rehabilitation.

Warm-up

Performing a warm-up prior to any form of exercise is a way of preparing your body and mind for exercise and sport. As the name suggests a warm-up increases your production of body heat and this heat is transported in the blood. As a result the blood vessels close to the surface of the skin will dilate and give you that healthy glowing appearance. The warmer blood will also be diverted to your skeletal muscles to provide them with the oxygen and nutrients needed for exercise. In addition to the heat transferred from the blood, the muscles themselves act as biochemical furnaces that generate the heat locally, and the heated muscles become more pliable and able to stretch. The effect is that the skeletal muscles and their tendons are primed for physical activity.

In order to get the extra blood to the working muscles the heart begins to beat faster and so the cardiovascular system is also readied for the exercise session. You will also notice the lungs breathing deeper and more frequently to get the extra oxygen in to the system. These actions ensure the exercising body will receive the required substances for producing the extra energy that is needed, and that waste products made by the working muscles are removed from the system.

The effects described above affect the body generally. More local effects, depending on the type of warm-up activity, will move the joints through a functional ROM. This ensures the structures around the joints are able to take the exercise stress. You should therefore choose your warm-up wisely. A gentle jog in circles may not be sufficient to adequately prepare the legs for lunges, and certainly will do little for getting the shoulders ready for push-ups or the inverted press. Instead of a jog you might want to consider some all-over movements that cover the body areas you intend to exercise. If you are not new to exercise and are already close to achieving the Seven Standards in this book then a variety of the preparatory exercises here-in may serve as an appropriate warm-up routine.

Finally, the act of warming-up will help focus your mind on the activity that is to come. It will hone the senses by redirecting blood flow. This can improve your motivation and focus, and these things can lead to a more productive and enjoyable workout.

To maximise the psychological effects of the warm-up you can set the scene by thinking through the routine you intend to do and visualise the exercises. Your physical environment will also help; so get your favourite exercise soundtrack on and get your mind in gear for each and every workout.

Clothing

If you are an exercise beginner it might seem like only the newest and trendiest clothes and workout gear are required to get results. Don't buy into the hype or marketing. No special clothes or footwear are needed for body weight exercise. If you want to look good then that is totally up to you. But if you *really* want to look good then you'll be the one doing all Seven Standards with perfect form, regardless of what you are wearing.

Our advice here is to wear something you are *comfortable* in - in terms of both the fit and the style. Ensure that the clothing allows the joints to move freely and that the compression around muscles does not hinder the flow of blood or their contraction. Your footwear should be well-fitted, have a stable sole, and be secure on your feet. If this is an expensive pair of trainers then that's fine, but if it's a cheap pair of pumps then that's fine too. Safety and comfort first! The style will shine through in your technique.

Our final note on clothing is to ensure you are able to properly regulate your body temperature. In the previous section we discussed how the body produces extra heat that is beneficial to getting the best out of your exercise session. However, if the body heat builds up because it is unable to escape then the body temperature will rise to dangerous levels. This can lead to heat stress and heat exhaustion and the effects can be fatal if prolonged. On the other end of the scale make sure you wear enough clothes in colder environments. If the body cools during exercise then it becomes less efficient and you may increase your risk of musculoskeletal injuries. We therefore suggest wearing layers of clothing that can be easily removed or added as needed.

Location

Many people have busy lives involving travel for work or family, and as such exercise can take place in many different locations. Exercise may take place at the gym, at home or in a home gym, hotels, and even outdoors.

As body weight exercise requires minimal specialist or expensive equipment, you should be fine performing the exercises in this book anywhere and at anytime. There are some pieces of equipment that are needed for some of the later exercises, but even these can be objects found around you such as exercise or playing equipment in parks. Much of the equipment needed to complete the exercises in the book can also be purchased widely at low cost.

In terms of your own exercise location, it should be somewhere that inspires you to train, and to reach the fitness and health goals you have set for yourself. If you dread going to the location where you will exercise then you will simply not go, and your health and fitness will not improve. This is the case whether the place you exercise is at home or at a gym; if the location is not inviting and motivating then you will be less likely to go!

9. Equipment

Although we love the fact that body weight exercise requires minimal equipment, there are some pieces of kit that make it easier to perform some of the higher-level movements. In this section we are going to take a brief look at some of this equipment. We'll give you tips and potential alternatives (if possible), and we'll also advise you on what to look out for and how best to use it.

Pull-up Bar

A pull-up bar is an essential piece of body weight exercise apparatus that allows you to maximise the resistance of gravity and body mass. Pull-up bars can be found in almost any good gym, and they can also be purchased for home use. The criteria that you should look for in this apparatus are: 1) a bar thickness that is comfortable to hold (too thick and it will be difficult to hold onto; too thin and the hands will pinch); 2) a suitable height from the ground, enabling easy and safe access; and 3) a sturdy point of attachment, ensuring your safety.

If you do not have a pull-up bar in your gym, or if you train from home, there are other options available. Pull-up bars for home use are now quite popular, with choices for many different situations. One option is to use a pull-up bar that secures to the doorframe, requiring no screws or bolts of any kind. If this is too temporary, it is possible to fix a pull-up bar to a wall or ceiling (but these obviously require a location that allows this, such as a basement or garage). Another option is a stand-alone unit that has a base and frame that support the bar; these types often come with dip bars as part of the structure, and so they can be a good investment (and are often cheaper than even a six-month gym membership). Alternatively, look for suitable fixed objects that can be found in many parks, which would also allow you to train outdoors.

Dip Bars

Dip bars are used for performing triceps dips. In the gym environment you will find two types; one is a simple two bar set-up, where two bars sit parallel to each other, around one and a half to two feet apart. The other type of dip bars are those found on an assisted machine (that normally comes with a pull-up station as well), that allows you to add weight to a moving platform that assists you with the exercise. These are preferable for the fact that you can vary the load to suit your needs, and are great for progressing with your triceps dips. The downside is that you will only find these in a gym environment.

Using proper dip bars for the triceps dip exercise is the ideal situation, but as we are huge fans of working out from home and not relying too much on equipment, it is worth exploring some alternative set-ups. The most obvious and easily accessible alternative is the backs of two chairs, as long as they are sturdy enough to hold your weight and will not tip over. You can use them just as you would normal triceps dip bars, to great effect. Other options are kitchen worktops (if they are close enough and will support your weight), boxes, or even walls that are close enough together and at the same height. Some parks or outdoor exercise spaces have parallel bars that are ideal for dip exercises.

Exercise Mat

Exercise mats, or yoga mats, are very useful for those movements that require the hands, elbows, or knees to be in contact with the floor. Some people at first may experience sore wrists, hands, or knees when their body is supported on the ground, and mats can help to lessen this effect. Any type of mat will do, as long as it is non-slip, and thick enough to adequately cushion the hands, elbows, or knees.

Exercise Step

The exercise step is most useful when adjusting the difficulty of some of the exercises like the push-up, for example. In raising or lowering the hands (or other parts of the body), weight can be moved away or towards the target muscles and joints, making the exercise in question easier or more difficult. With the example of the push-up, raising the hands moves more weight onto the lower body, making the exercise easier.

Exercise steps can be found in all gyms around the world, but these are not the only things that can be used for this purpose. Stairs, the edges of couches, the edges of chairs, sturdy boxes, and other similar objects can all be used in this way. The only requirement is that it is able to safely support your body weight.

10. The Seven Standards

Now that you have some background knowledge of body weight exercise it is time to learn the exercises that make up the Seven Standards of body weight exercise. Don't be daunted by these standards - they are challenging, but they are achievable. Sitting behind each Standard are six preparatory exercises that are of varying difficulty and will help you develop the physical attributes necessary for each of the Standards. That's a total of seven exercises in each of the Seven Standards. We have broken each exercise down to make it as straightforward as possible to follow.

Firstly we justify our choice of exercise and then outline some basic anatomy. We want you to understand why you are doing each exercise, its benefits, and the parts of your body being targeted. The latter will help you better appreciate your post-exercise aches (see the section on DOMS).

The next section asks the question: *Where To Do It*. Here we explain what sort of equipment you might need (if any), and anything else you might need to know before actually doing the exercise.

The third section is *How To Do It*, and explains clearly how to perform the exercise. We also supplement the description with photographic illustration.

The fourth section is our *Teaching Points*. Here we address issues that might arise when performing the exercise, and how to correct them. This could include some common errors or some guidance on how to modify the exercise to better suit your current abilities.

The final section is *When To Progress*, and helps you decide when to progress from a preparatory exercise to the Standard, or beyond!

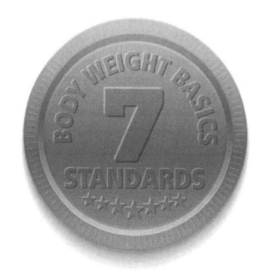

10.1 Standard One: The Push-up

The push-up is perhaps the most well-known of all body weight exercises. When it comes to developing upper-body strength the push-up is probably the most executed of all conditioning exercises. It forms the bedrock of many military training programmes and is the staple of those attempting a basic fitness in their own homes.

Though it is a very popular body weight exercise, we have recognised that in our experience few people can perform a single push-up with good technique (form). The perfect push-up will be controlled and not jerky, and will have a good depth of movement. The posture should ideally be relaxed through the neck and shoulders, with a tight abdomen and neutral spine aligned with taut buttocks and thighs. Who would have thought so much was going on in this most fundamental of body weight exercises?

There are many ways to perform push-ups incorrectly, but there are few ways to do the ideal technique. Achieving perfect form is not an easy task but you got this book because you wanted a challenge. You wanted to improve your basic strength and physical ability. To help you in your challenge we will share with you the preparatory exercises that we feel develop the key elements of the push-up. We will demonstrate how the push-up can be simplified and regressed to the point that anyone can achieve the basics, from which point you can develop the picture-perfect push-up.

Before identifying the model technique let us first look at the muscles and joints being targeted with the push-up.

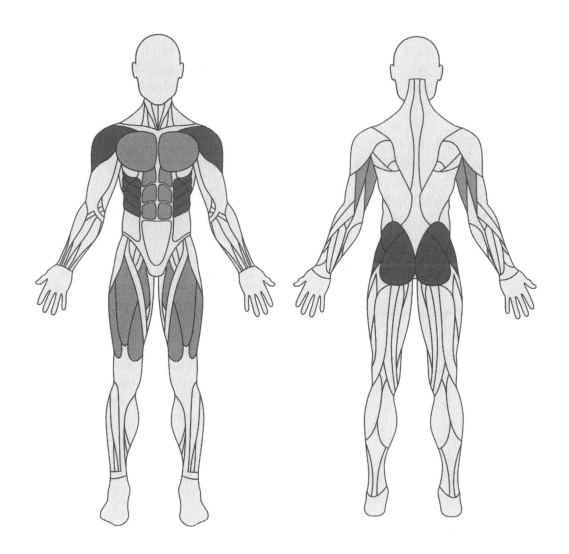

FIGURE 1.1. The Anatomy of the Push-up: Pectoralis major, anterior deltoids, triceps, rectus abdominus, transverus abdominus, gluteus maximus, and quadriceps.

As the push-up is so well-recognized and practiced you will probably already know that it is used as an exercise for building the chest muscles. Predominantly it is the pectoralis major muscles that are strengthened with push-ups; a pair of muscles sitting on the front of the upper rib cage, as can be seen in Figure 1.1.

The 'Pecs' as they are often referred to pass from the chest to the top of the upper arm bone (humerus). In the push-up position the pecs contract to draw the upper arm bone towards the midline of the body. This single movement of 'horizontal adduction' is the key to the press-up action. The movement comes from the shoulder joint and so the pecs are assisted in this exercise by the large shoulder muscles – the deltoids (Figure 1.1).

When the shoulders move during the push-up the elbow joints must also allow movement to bring the chest away from the ground. The elbows straighten (extend) to drive the body upwards during a push-up and this requires the triceps muscles to contract. We can therefore add another muscle to our first body weight workout - the triceps at the back of the upper arm (Figure 1.1).

Finally, in order to maintain the trunk and leg alignment during the push-up the following muscles are used:

• Abdominal muscle groups (rectus abdominus and transverus abdominus); to stop the lower spine sagging.
• Gluteus maximus; to prevent the hips and pelvis collapsing
• Quadriceps muscle group, to maintain a straight (extended) knee

Where the pectoralis major, deltoid, and triceps muscles all change length whilst contracting, the muscles listed above work 'isometrically'. This means that when they contract during the push-up they keep the same length to stabilise rather than move the trunk. These stability muscles are shown in Figure 1.1.

Now that we have an appreciation of what muscles and joints contribute to the push-up we can take a look at the desired technique.

Key Features Of The Push-Up

Some key features of the push-up are as follows:

• Shoulders should remain over the hands at all times
• Core should remain tight
• Head and neck should remain neutral
• The shoulders, hips, and feet should form a straight line
• Arms begin straight, with no bend in the elbow
• Chest should touch the ground on every repetition

Performing The Push-up

The first Body weight Basics Standard is one of the most popular and well recognised body weight exercises that exists. Read on to find out exactly how to effectively perform the first Standard.

Where To Do It

You will require some floor space and a mat for your knees if needed.

How To Do It

1. Place both hands on the ground, fingers facing forwards, hands shoulder width apart.

2. Stretch your legs out behind you and balance on your toes.

3. Raise your hips up until your shoulders, hips, and feet form a straight line.

4. Keeping your head and neck in a neutral position, bend your elbows and begin lowering your chest towards the ground.

5. Allow your elbows to flare out to the sides slightly, and descend until your chest or torso touches the ground. Keep the neck in a neutral position, trying not to let your head fall forwards.

6. Pause for a second, and then push back up again, keeping the body straight.

7. Return to the start position, with the elbows straight. This counts as one repetition.

Teaching Points

There are a number of Teaching Points to consider with the push-up.

First, there may be a lack of strength or mobility to allow the chest to reach the ground. This will improve with graded exercise practice. The following preparatory exercises will gradually take you through a progressive range and degree of resistance to build your joint range and muscle strength.

Second, you may struggle keeping a neutral neck position throughout the movement. A common fault is to allow the head to bob forward. To address this, keep your eyes fixed on a spot on the ground between your hands, with the neck muscles loose and relaxed.

Third, the angle to which the elbows flare out may fluctuate: if they are too close to your torso then the chest muscles will not be involved enough and you will find the exercise more difficult. If they are too far away from your torso the push-up will feel awkward and you will not be able to push as strongly.

When To Progress

The goal with the push-up is to be able to perform 8 repetitions, with perfect form. When you can do this you will have mastered one of the Seven Standards!

To help you master the first of the Seven Standards of Body Weight Basics we have gathered together a set of preparatory exercises that will help in developing the necessary strength and function. These exercises are presented in the following sections, starting with the kneeling platform push-up.

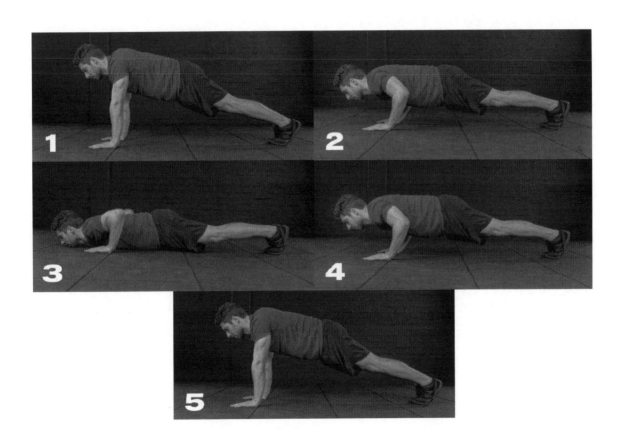

Kneeling Platform Push-up

The first stage in learning the push-up is to strip back the exercise and make it as simple as possible. This allows first time exercisers, and those who are deconditioned, to take part and progress. The easiest version of the push-up is the kneeling platform push-up. This is where the hands are placed on a raised platform, and the lower body is supported on the knees. Placing the hands on the platform reduces the resistance created by body weight, as the lower body is supported on the knees. The height of the platform will vary the difficulty of the exercise. A higher platform makes the exercise easier, and a lower platform makes the exercise harder.

Where To Do It

You will need a platform of some kind to perform the kneeling platform push-up. This can be a set of stairs, an exercise box or step, the edge of a sofa or bed, or anything else that is sturdy and at the height of your knees when standing. If you have something that can be adjusted in height then that is better, as you can adjust the difficulty of the exercise!

How To Do It

1. Kneel down in front of the platform and let your feet rest on the ground. If you have sore knees then use a mat to cushion them. You may have to adjust the distance between the platform and your knees depending on your height, and how high the platform is that you are using.

2. Place your hands on the platform, with your hands shoulder width apart, fingers splayed slightly and pointing forwards.

3. Make sure that your thighs and torso form a straight line, and that your head is in a neutral position. Do not allow your head to drop or strain to one side.

4. Start to bend your elbows and lower your chest towards your hands. Allow your elbows to move out as much as you need them to, in whatever direction is comfortable.

5. Keep going until your chest either touches the platform, or you reach the limit of your strength or mobility.

6. Pause for a second, and then push back up under control. Aim to breathe out whilst doing the return effort. This is one repetition.

Teaching Points

Common issues with the kneeling push-up include moving the head excessively and straining the neck, and letting the hips drop and the low-back sag. We would refer to these issues as problems with your 'form'. These could reduce the effectiveness of the exercise or may even increase your risk of injury. Make sure that you keep your head neutral, tighten your core muscles, and take it slowly. If you find that you are struggling, then raise the height of the platform until you can do the kneeling push-up correctly.

When To Progress

Move on to the next stage when you can perform 8 reps with good form, using a platform that is 6-12 inches high.

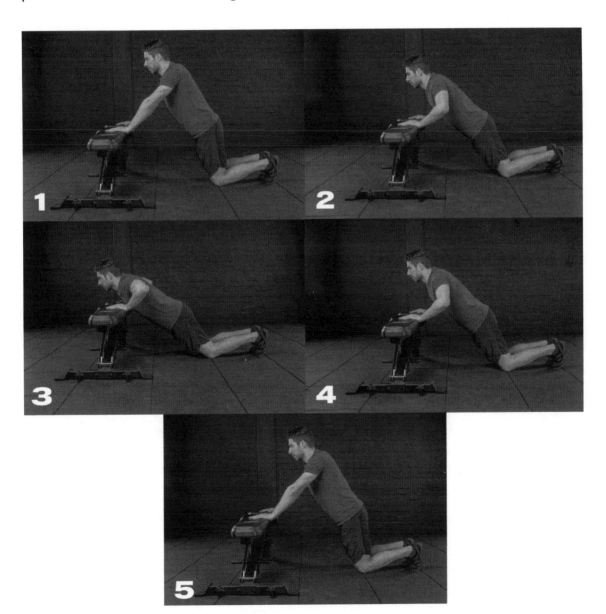

Kneeling Push-up

Once you have managed to gain some experience with the kneeling platform push-up, you should move onto the kneeling push-up. This is performed in exactly the same manner as the first variation, except that the hands will be placed on level ground rather than on a raised step.

Where To Do It

For the kneeling push-up all you will need is some level floor space and a mat for your knees (if you have knee pain). A cushioned or carpeted floor that is free of dust is recommended.

How To Do It

1. Kneel down on the floor and let your feet rest on the ground. If you have sore knees then use a mat to cushion them. A folded towel works well here.

2. Place your hands on the ground, with your hands shoulder width apart, fingers splayed slightly and pointing forwards. The load should be through the palms of the hand rather than the fingers.

3. Make sure that your thighs and torso form a straight line, and that your head is in a neutral position. Do not allow your head to drop or strain to one side.

4. Start to bend your elbows and lower your chest towards your hands. Allow your elbows to move out as much as you need them to, in whatever direction is comfortable. In most instance the upper arms will be at right-angles to the trunk of the body.

5. Keep going until your chest either touches the ground, or you reach the limit of your strength or mobility. Pause for a second, and then push back up under control. Aim to breathe out whilst doing the return effort. This is one repetition.

Teaching Points

One common problem when trying kneeling push-ups is lacking the flexibility or strength to allow the chest to reach the floor. Your flexibility will get better over time as you gradually develop the strength to safely control the movement, so keep practicing!

When To Progress

Move on from this stage when you can perform 8 reps, with your chest touching the ground on each rep, with good form.

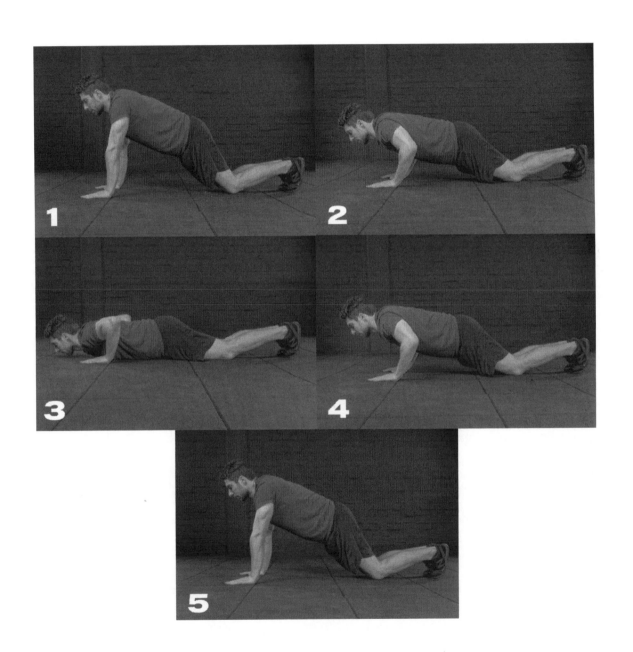

Platform Push-up

The third stage in developing the push-up is the platform push-up. This exercise uses a platform like preparatory exercise 1.1, but you will balance on your toes instead of your knees. The difficulty is changed in the same way; making the body more vertical (using a higher platform) makes the movement easier; making the body more horizontal (using a lower platform) makes the movement harder.

Where To Do It

For the platform push-up you can use the same platform as for the kneeling platform push-up (exercise 1.2), although if you prefer you can start with a much higher surface, such as the side of a worktop or table, or even a window-sill. Just make sure whatever you use will not move when you lean against it!

How To Do It

1. Get into a push-up position with your hands on the platform and your toes on the ground. Raise your hips from the ground so that your shoulders, chest, waist, and legs form a straight line. Ensure that your head is in a neutral position. Do not allow your head to drop or strain to one side.

2. Start to bend your elbows and lower your chest towards the platform. Allow your elbows to move out as much as you need them to, in whatever direction is comfortable. In most instances the upper arms will be at right-angles to the trunk of the body.

3. Keep going until your chest either touches the platform, or you reach the limit of your strength or mobility.

4. Pause for a second, and then push back up under control. Aim to breathe out whilst doing the return effort. This is one repetition.

Teaching Points

The main point to the platform push-up is that you can adjust the height of the platform to adjust the difficulty of the exercise. If you are struggling to perform the exercise correctly, or cannot achieve a big enough range of motion, then raise the platform height until you can. As you progress and get stronger, simply decrease the height of the platform!

When Do I Progress?

Move on to the next exercise when you can perform 8 reps with good form in a single set on a platform of 18 inches or less.

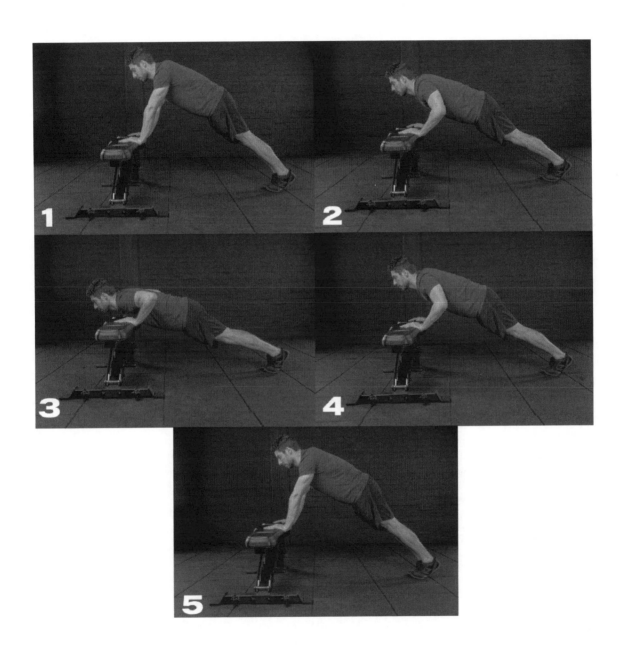

Negative Push-up

This stage in developing the push-up is an essential one, and is also the first time that you will use the negative phase of the movement to get stronger. The term *negative phase* sounds like jargon, but it simply means to *move with control in the direction of gravity.*

For the push-up, this means starting in the top position and then lowering yourself towards the ground as slowly as possible. This allows the muscles to be under tension as they lengthen, which builds greater strength than the positive (return) phase . Once you get to the floor you relax, and the repetition is complete. This may sound easy, but the idea is to go as slow as possible! Remember, with this exercise the slower the better.

Where To Do It

You will require some floor space, and a mat for your knees and chest when you reach the floor. We recommend a cushioned, padded or carpeted floor that is free of dust.

How To Do It

1. To perform the negative push-up, start in the top position of the push-up. Your hands should be flat on the ground, shoulder width apart, with your torso and legs in a straight line.

2. Balance on your toes and make sure that your entire body is taut. Your head should be in a neutral position. Your chest will ideally be aligned with your hands.

3. Bend your elbows and lower yourself towards the ground as slowly and controlled as possible.

4. Keep lowering yourself down until your chest reaches the floor. Now rest. This counts as one repetition. From here you can kneel up and reset the start position.

Teaching Points

A common issue with negative push-ups is being stronger at certain points of the exercise than others. For example, you may be very strong at the top of the movement, when there is only a small bend in the elbows. But, when the bend in the elbow starts to become greater your weakness will show and you will drop to the floor. Do your best to control that final part of the motion and the more you practice, the stronger you will get.

When To Progress

You should progress to the next stage when you take 15 seconds to go from the top position to the ground, whilst keeping good form in your body and head posture. Aim to complete three consecutive sets of this.

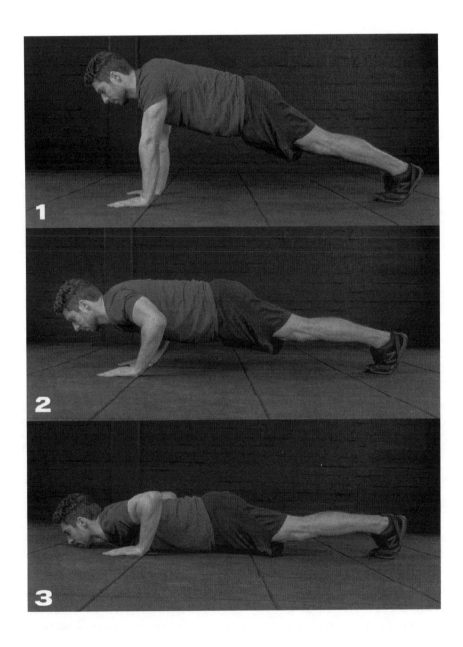

Static Hold Push-up

As well as the negative type of movement there is the static type as well. *Static* means to stay still, and that is exactly what this exercise is all about. To do this preparatory exercise you will get into a push-up position with your elbows bent, and then try and hold that position for as long as possible. This means that your muscles will be contracting but staying the same length. This is great for building strength, and also for building mental stamina and determination.

Where To Do It

You will need some floor space and a mat for your knees (if you have sore joints). We recommend a cushioned, padded or carpeted floor that is free of dust.

How To Do It

1. Get into a push-up position. Your hands should be flat on the ground, shoulder width apart, and you should be balancing on your toes, with legs straight and hips in line with the shoulders and feet.

2. Bend your elbows until they have a 90-degree bend in them.

3. Hold this position as long as possible, and then gently drop onto your knees and rest when you can hold no longer. This counts as one repetition.

Teaching Points

You may find that you lack the strength to hold the position with a 90-degree bend in the elbow. If this is the case try a smaller bend in the elbow, such as 45 degrees, or even 30 degrees. As you get stronger you will be able to hold the position with a greater bend in the elbow.

Another potential issue is a lack of core strength, which will mean that your hips and low-back start to sag before your chest and arms tire. Work with the plank (Body weight Standard 6) to improve your core strength.

When To Progress

You should progress to the next stage when you can hold the push-up position with a 90-degree bend in the elbow for 30 seconds, whilst maintaining good posture in the body and head. Aim to complete three consecutive sets of this.

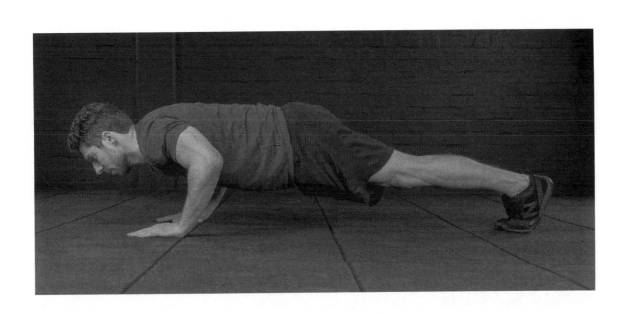

Shallow Push-up

Now that you are familiar with the basic elements of the push-up, this preparatory exercise is about putting it all together. We call this the shallow push-up. In effect, you will be performing a push-up but with a reduced range of motion. Starting at the top, you will bend your elbows a small amount, before pushing back up to the start position. This method allows a huge range of abilities to actually practice the push-up motion without dropping to the ground.

Where To Do It

All you need to perform the shallow push-up is some floor space, and a mat to protect against sore knees. We recommend a cushioned, padded or carpeted floor that is free of dust.

How To Do It

1. To perform the shallow push-up, get into the top push-up position. Your hands should be flat on the ground, shoulder width apart, balancing on your toes, with legs straight and hips in line with the shoulder and feet.

2. Bend your elbows slightly and allow them to flare out to the sides, at around 45 degrees.

3. Keep bending your elbows until you feel resistance, then push back up to the top again. Depending on your abilities this may be a few inches, or you may even achieve a 90-degree bend in your elbow. Regardless of your level, make sure that you can push back up to the top position, whilst holding the form in your trunk and neck. This is one repetition.

Teaching Points

When doing the shallow push-up do not introduce too much range of motion too soon. This exercise is designed to be shallow, so that you can perform 5 to 10 reps without dropping to the ground and without going to failure. It will help develop endurance in the muscles described at the start of this Standard: The Push-Up. To begin with, only lower yourself down a small distance, and build from there.

When To Progress

To progress to the net stage, you should be able to perform 8 reps, with your elbows bending to at least 90 degrees on each rep, but not more than 90 degrees. Aim to complete three consecutive sets of this.

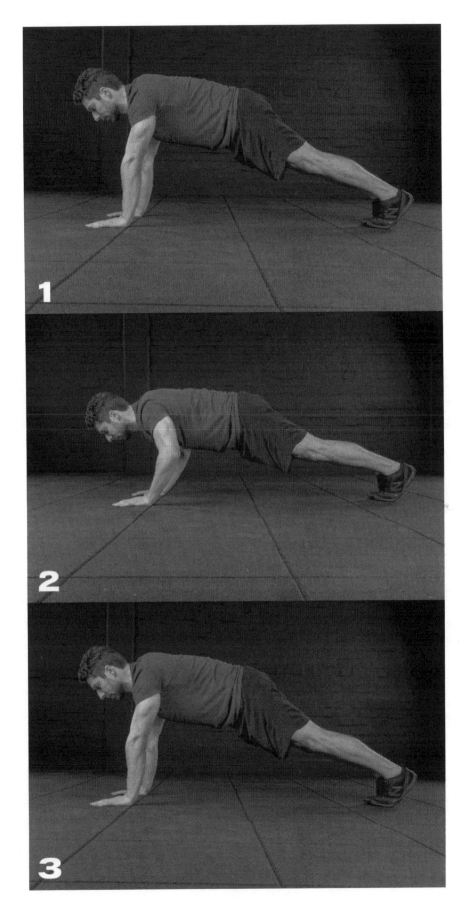

10.2 Standard Two: The Pull-up

If the push-up is one of the most well-known body weight exercises then the pull-up is probably one of the most desirable. Most people would want to be able to do one (or more!) but in reality few people can. This is also in contrast to the push-up we reviewed in Standard One, where most people can do at least one push-up in some form or another (usually with less-than-ideal form). The pull-up however has to overcome the resistance of nearly all of your body weight. This makes our Standard Two of the Body Weight Basics programme perhaps the toughest, and therefore the most rewarding achievement of the whole book. Forget muscle-ups and one-handed pull-ups; if you can develop your physical strength to achieve three pull-ups with perfect form then you have earned our respect.

So why is the pull-up so difficult? Firstly, as discussed, it requires you to overcome the resistance of almost all of your body weight. There are three broad ways to achieve this: 1) learn an efficient technique, 2) get stronger, 3) lose body weight if carrying excess. This book deals with the first two points in the following preparatory exercises. The third point is beyond the scope of this book but if you are carrying excess body weight then we recommend you seek professional advice and support to help with this. Losing excess weight will help in your Body weight Basics goals and may also have numerous other health and fitness benefits.

Secondly, all of your body weight is hanging below your hands meaning that you need to develop a good grip. This element should not be taken for granted as it is a fundamental component of many more progressive body weight exercises. The good news is that you can develop your hanging grip with the following preparatory exercises.

But before we get to the preparatory exercises, let's look at the major joints and muscles required to perform the pinnacle of body weight exercises – the pull-up.

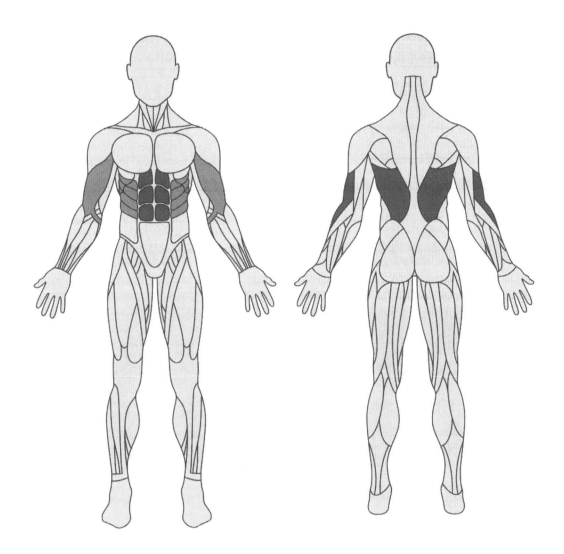

FIGURE 2.1: The Anatomy of the Pull-up: Latissimus dorsi, biceps, brachioradialis, rectus abdominis and transversus abdominis.

When you see the pull-up being performed it is often obvious to note the muscles being targeted. In a well-trained individual you may see the broad back muscles that fan out from the middle-spine towards the armpits and then taper down to the low-spine and pelvis to create the inverted triangular shape.

These are the latissimus dorsi muscles, as shown in Figure 2.1. Like the pectoralis major muscles featured in Standard One: The Push-Up, the latissimus dorsi muscles cross from the trunk to the upper part of the upper arm bone (humerus). When the arm is raised above head-height the 'lats', as they are more commonly known, are perfectly positioned on a slight stretch to pull the arm back toward the sides of the body. This is the essence of the pull-up, only the action is reversed and it is the body that is being pulled up to be reunited with arms.

When you see the pull-up in action you can also see that the elbows bend (flex). This movement against resistance requires the contraction of the biceps muscles of the upper arm. The biceps are shown in Figure 2.1. This again contrasts nicely with Standard One: The Push-up that works the triceps muscle at the back of the upper arm in order to create elbow extension. The push-up and the pull-up therefore provide balance to resistance training of the upper body and arms.

In Body Weight Basics we emphasise the over-hand grip with a reasonably wide hand spacing, as can be seen in the following section on the mechanics of the pull-up. The pull-up can also be performed with a narrower over-hand grip or even a 'hammer' grip. These variations will also recruit another muscle at the elbow called brachioradialis, also shown in Figure 2.1. Pull-ups can also be performed with an under-hand grip to further develop the biceps but these are technically referred to as 'chin-ups' and do not feature in the book. Instead we focus on the more rewarding 'pull-up'.

Finally, in order to stop the spine from over-arching during the pull-up the abdominal muscle groups are recruited to keep a tight and stable trunk. Figure 2.1 shows the abdominal muscles - the rectus abdominis and transversus abdominis.

Key Features Of The Pull-Up

Some key features of the pull-up are as follows:

• Elbows should be straight and body relaxed to start
• Grip should be slightly wider than shoulder width
• Legs and core should remain still during the pull phase
• Chin should rise above the bar
• Ideally, the chest will touch the bar
• Each rep should be performed with control

Performing The Pull-up

Continuing our examination of this Standard, we are going to show you how to perform the pull-up. This will give you an idea of what it takes to master this Standard. This is a very difficult exercise to master so allow yourself time and focus on the fundamentals. With time you will see great gains in strength and physique.

Where To Do It

You will need a pull-up bar (or similar) that is positioned preferably just above your reaching height, so that you can relax your legs beneath you without touching the floor.

How To Do It

1. Grab the pull-up bar with both hands in an overgrip position (palms facing forwards).

2. Hang from the bar, with torso and legs straight, head in a neutral position.

3. Pull down with your shoulders so that they move away from your ears. This will help activate the necessary muscles and prevent shoulder strain.

4. Begin to pull yourself towards the bar, keeping your legs relaxed. Use the arms and back muscles to raise yourself towards the bar rather than using using momentum from your legs and trunk.

5. Keep going until your chin is over the bar (minimum requirement), or your chest touches the bar (ideal requirement).

6. Pause for a second, and then lower yourself down to the start position. This counts as one repetition.

Teaching Points

Of all of the exercises in this book the pull-up is the one that may provide the biggest challenge. We understand this as we have spent many hours mastering the pull-up. From our experience we provide a few pointers to make your journey easier.

First, do not rush the preparatory exercises outlined in the next sections. Move on to Standard Two when you are ready and have developed the necessary strength and control. If you move too quickly then you will not have built the basics required to perform a proper pull-up.

Second, do not cheat! Make sure that your arms are fully straight when you reach the bottom position, and do not be tempted to kick or lift the legs when pulling up. Keep momentum to a minimum when developing strength and control.

Lastly, squeeze the bar firmly. This will help to focus your strength. A loose grip can also cause hand and wrist problems.

When To Progress

The aim with Standard Two: The Pull-up is to be able to perform 3 perfect reps, one after the other. This will take some effort, but is well worth it! Good luck!

To help you master this Standard we have gathered together a set of preparatory exercises that will help in developing the necessary strength and function. These exercises are presented in the following sections, starting with the standing row.

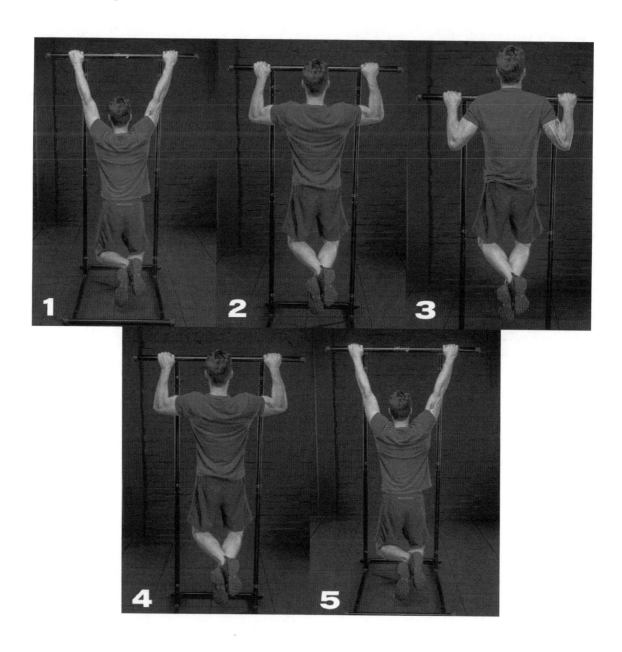

Standing Row

So, how do you begin to learn the pull-up? As with every exercise in this book, the movement itself needs to be stripped down to its component parts. The first stage to learning the pull-up is the standing row. This preparatory exercise will familiarize your body with the pulling motion, and will begin to work the muscles that are responsible for the pull-up.

Where To Do It

You will need a bar for the standing row, preferably one that is at shoulder height, and preferably one that is adjustable. Most gyms will have something like this that you can use. In fact, one of the best pieces of equipment for this exercise is the Smith machine. This is an apparatus where the bar can be adjusted in height, allowing you to progress the row by altering the height of the bar. If you do not have access to a gym then you can improvise by holding the edges of an open door frame. This will require a different grip so please go steady at first.

How To Do It

1. To perform the standing row, face the bar and grab it with both hands, palms facing towards the floor. Your feet should be positioned directly underneath the bar.

2. Lean back until your arms are straight. Your legs and torso should form a straight line, and your body should be at an angle, so that if you let go of the bar you would fall over. Don't let go of the bar!

3. Pull on the bar and lever yourself over your planted feet, until your chest touches the bar, or you cannot pull any further. Keep your body straight and maintain a neutral position of the head and neck. If using the door frame as an improvisation then bring yourself upright so that your chest meets the space between the door frame.

4. Pause for a second, then return slowly to the start position. This counts as one repetition.

Teaching Points

Beware of simple errors and bad habits that can hinder your progress. Make sure that your entire body is straight, and that your torso and legs from a straight line. Second, keep your feet planted on the ground and wear footwear that prevents the feet from slipping.

When To Progress

When you can perform 8 reps easily, with your torso and legs straight, then you can move on to the next stage.

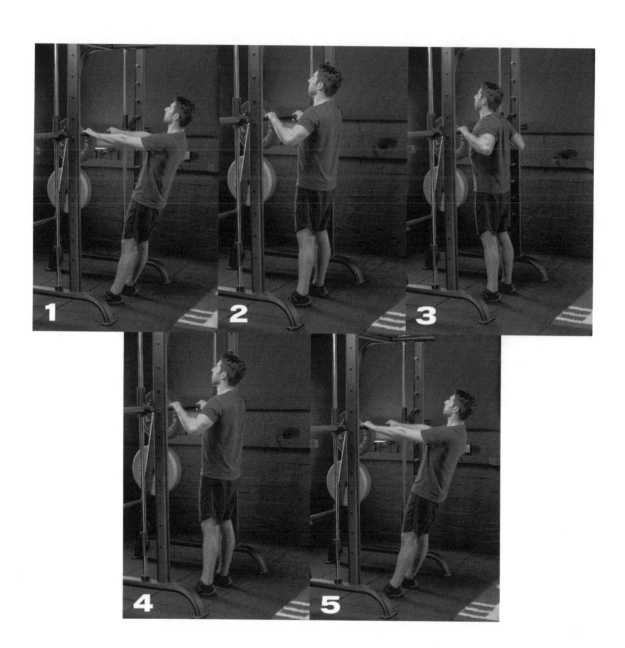

Supine Row

When you can perform the standing row (Preparatory exercise 2.1) with ease you can start to change the angle of your body to increase the difficulty. This exercise is called the supine row. Supine means 'face up'. The movement is the same as the standing row, except that the body will be held at a shallower angle. Where the feet were positioned directly under the bar in the standing row, for the supine row the feet should be moved forward of this position, so that the body becomes more horizontal. You may therefore feel it is easier to rest on your heels. The more horizontal the body position, the more difficult the exercise will be. This is because more load (body weight) is pulling under the bar. This ability to alter the body position allows the difficulty of the exercise to be altered in line with your abilities.

Where To Do It

You can use the same bar and set-up for the supine row as you did with the standing row. The only difference is that the bar should be set lower, and be adjusted down towards waist height. The improvised exercise suggested for exercise 2.1 will be less appropriate here. Instead try lying under a table and gripping the sides of the table to suspend yourself above the floor. Ensure the table is stable and can support your weight.

How To Do It

1. To perform the supine row stand in front of the bar and grab it with both hands. Your grip should be shoulder width apart, and your palms should be facing downwards.

2. Position your feet under the bar to start with (the same as with the standing row) then move them forward until you are suspended about 45 degrees to the horizontal.

3. Pull on the bar until your chest touches it, or you cannot pull any further. Keep your body straight and head in a neutral position. If doing the improvised version using a table then pull until your chin gently reaches the underside of the table.

4. Pause for a second, and then return to the starting position. This counts as one repetition.

Teaching Points

To make the exercise harder, move the feet forward to make the body more horizontal. To make the exercise easier, move the feet backward to make the body more vertical.

When To Progress

When you can perform 8 reps with your body angled at 45 degrees and maintaining good form, then move onto the next stage.

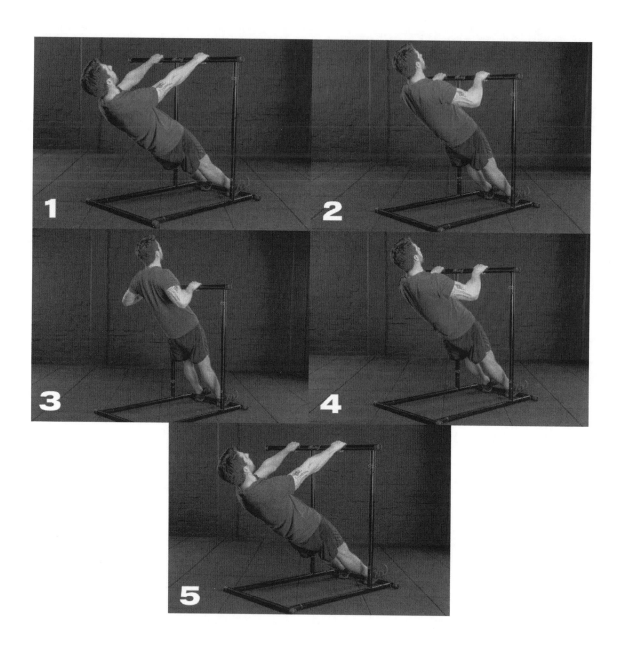

Dead Hang

After you have progressed from preparatory exercises 2.1 and 2.2 then it will be time to get to grips with an actual pull-up bar, literally! This exercise might seem trivial, but being able to hang on a bar and support your own body weight is essential to being able to perform a pull-up. If you cannot support your own body weight when hanging from a bar, you will stand little chance of pulling yourself toward that bar.

Where To Do It

You will need access to a high horizontal bar of some kind, preferably one that is not too high, and that you can reach without jumping. This could be a pull-up bar in a gym, one that can be easily purchased and fixed in a door frame at home, or the frame of a child's swing (or similar).

With a bar of sufficient height you will be able to tuck your legs up to initiate the dead hang, instead of jumping and grabbing a bar. This will keep you safe and prevent a drop to the floor once you have finished the exercise.

How To Do It

1. To perform the dead hang grab a pull-up bar with an overhand grip. Your hands should be slightly wider than shoulder width apart.

2. Make sure that your elbows are straight and your head is in a neutral position.

3. Now lift your feet off the ground, either by bending the knees or tucking up your thighs to your stomach.

4. Simply hang onto the bar for as long as possible. Concentrate on squeezing the bar, using your hands and forearms to develop a strong grip.

5. As soon as you start to feel your grip loosen, or feel that you are going to drop off the bar, then lower yourself to the floor and rest. This counts as one set.

Teaching Points

Initially you may develop sore hands if your skin is not used to the pressure being placed upon it. In this instance you can use exercise gloves, chalk, or gymnastic bar grips to ease the pull on the skin. Eventually the palms of the hand may callous slightly. With the dead hang avoid bending the elbows. This exercise is about developing hanging ability, and that includes the stretch gained around the shoulders and back muscles.

When To Progress

Move onto the next stage when you can perform a dead hang for 30 seconds.

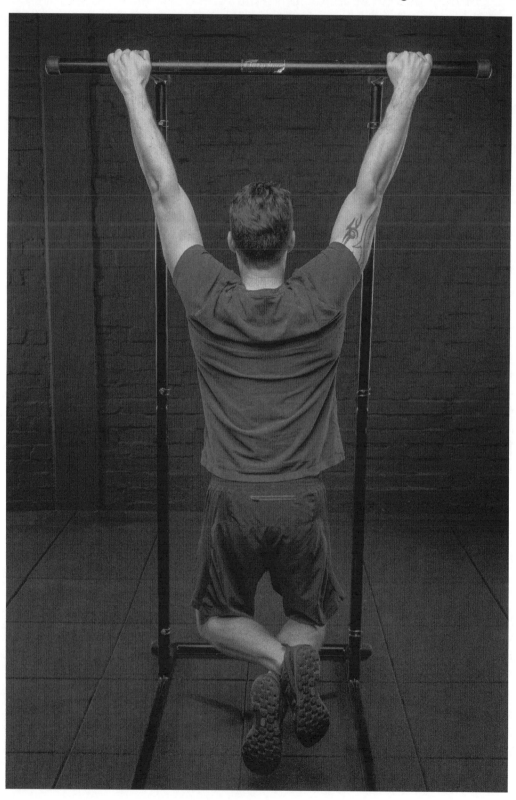

Pull-up Pulses

Once you can perform the dead hang (exercise 2.3) for at least 30 seconds it will be time to move onto the fourth preparatory exercise in this section - pull-up pulses. This exercise combines the dead hang and a very small pulling motion. The idea behind this exercise is to build strength in the very bottom part of the movement. This is where the elbows go from completely straight to slightly bent, and it is the hardest part of the pull-up where inertia is greatest.

Believe it or not, this small range of motion at the bottom of the pull-up position is where most people cheat on pull-ups. It is extremely tempting to only drop down to where the arms are slightly bent, as this makes the exercise easier. But you got this book because you want to do a proper pull-up, so read on!

Where To Do It

You will need a pull-up bar of some kind, preferably one that you can grab on tiptoe.

How To Do It

1. Grab a pull-up bar with both hands in an overhand grip, hands slightly wider than shoulder width apart.

2. Get into a dead hang, so that your feet are not touching the ground. See exercise 2.3 to remind yourself of this position.

3. Now pull up slightly, just enough so that you elbows bend by a few degrees. Try not to cheat by thrusting yourself upwards. Generate as much of the pull from your arms as possible.

4. Repeat for 5 reps.

Teaching Points

You may find pull-up pulses deceptively difficult, but this is OK! They are meant to be tough otherwise you would never get stronger. Concentrate on the lowest part of the pull-up movement, and try and get a very small bend at the elbow. This 'break away' force is essential to being able to do full pull-ups with good form.

When To Progress

Move onto the next stage when you can perform 10 pull-up pulses in one set.

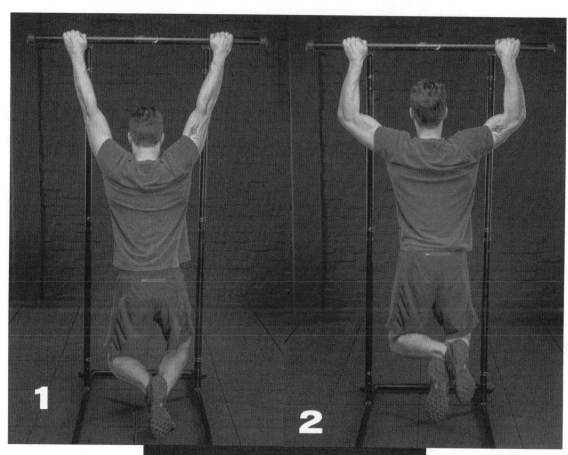

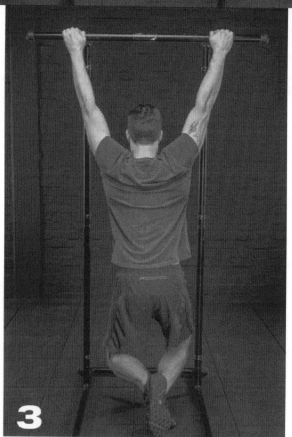

Negative Pull-up

Now that you have mastered the dead hang (preparatory exercise 2.4), and have some experience with the pulling motion, it is time to use the power of gravity to increase your strength. Negative pull-ups are where you start at the top of the movement and allow gravity to pull you down to earth, whilst trying to lower yourself slowly. This method is one of the best for increasing strength in the biceps and back muscles.

Where To Do It

You will need access to a pull-up bar or similar (as outlined earlier in this section), and enough space below and behind for you to drop off the bar when needed. You will also need a step or platform of some kind, to allow you to start the exercise with your chin at the level of the bar.

How To Do It

1. Grab the pull-up bar with both hands in an overhand grip, hands slightly wider than shoulder width apart.

2. Step onto the platform and stand up straight, so that your chin is either level with the bar or over it (if your bar is low then you may be able to stand on the floor and get into this position).

3. Contract your muscles hard and pull on the bar to take your own weight. This will feel hard. Lift your feet off the platform (or ground if your bar is low) and hold yourself in place.

4. Start to lower yourself as slowly as possible. Pull on the bar and gradually let your muscles lengthen as gravity pulls you down.

5. Keep going all the way until your arms are completely straight, then drop off or let go of the bar, and rest. This counts as one repetition.

Teaching Points

The most common problem seen with this exercise is the different levels of strength people have at different stages. For example, at the top of the movement you may feel very strong, as your muscles are shortened, but towards the bottom you may feel weaker. At the top you may move slowly and be well-controlled while at the bottom you may move quickly. The only way to get better is to practice, and in time your strength will increase.

When To Progress

Move onto the next stage when it takes you 15 seconds to go from the top position of the pull-up to the bottom position of the pull-up.

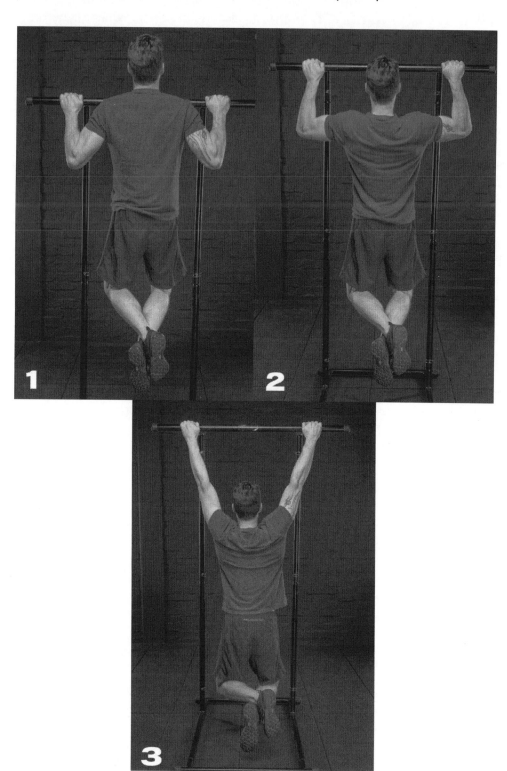

Assisted Pull-up

Congratulations! If you are at this stage then you are close to achieving a pull-up. This stage involves working with the full version of the pull-up! The assisted version can be done in a number of ways, but the best and most effective is with an assisted pull-up machine. This will allow you to make steady progress and adjust the difficulty.

Failing this you will need a partner who can provide some support by cupping under your bent knees to offload some body weight. Another alternative is to purchase some elastic therapy band and loop a long length around the bar to provide a sling that you can cradle your knees in. These bands comes in different strengths (and colours) and so can provide variable amounts of support. Please ensure you tie the knot tightly if using this equipment and that the band is free of tears or defects.

Where To Do It

Ideally you should have access to an assisted pull-up machine. These can be found in most gyms, and work in the opposite way to most weights machines. On assisted machines, the more weight you add the easier the exercise becomes. Alternatively, see our recommendations above.

How To Do It

1. First, set up the machine with enough weight so that you can comfortably perform the movement and will not get stuck. For example, if you weigh 80 kg (180 lbs) then make sure the machine is loaded with at least 50% of this weight (40 kg, or 90 lbs).

2. Now get into position. This will depend on the type of machine you have access to, but your hands should grip the bar in an overhand grip, hands slightly wider than shoulder width apart. Your knees or feet should rest on the support pad, and your entire torso should be vertical.

3. Lower yourself to the bottom position. Your arms should be straight, with no bend in the elbow. Your legs and torso should also be in line, as vertical as you can get them.

4. Now start to pull up, gripping the bar tightly, and bringing your elbows to your sides. Keep going until your chin is level with the bar, pause for a second, and then reverse the movement until you arrive at the bottom again. This counts as one repetition.

Teaching Points

To progress with the assisted pull-up reduce the amount of assistance that the machine gives you a little at a time. Don't be tempted to drop the amount of weight on the machine by many kilograms or pounds at a time; try 5 kg or 10 lbs every few weeks, until you are comfortable at that new weight. This way you will build strength progressively and safely. If using alternative methods of assistance, such as the therapy elastic bands, use either a thinner band or make a longer loop with less tension in. Both of these will place more stress on your arms and back. If using a partner for assistance then have them support you under your shins instead of at the knees.

When To Progress

You should move onto the next stage when you can do 5 reps with 20% of your body weight on the machine. For example, if you weigh 80 kg (180 lbs), then you will need to be able to do 5 reps with 16 kg (36 lbs) on the machine. This means you are lifting 80% of your own weight. On the alternative methods we have suggested you will need to estimate this amount based on the effort.

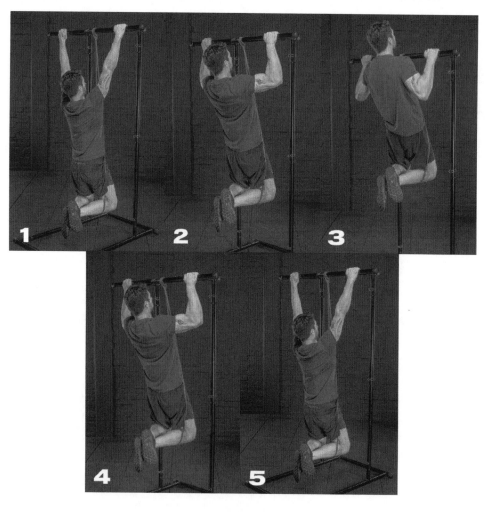

10.3 Standard Three: The Triceps Dip

There are no prizes for guessing what muscle is being worked here (*triceps* - in case you guessed incorrectly!), but don't be fooled into thinking it is the only muscle being worked in this Standard. Like all the body weight exercises we have gathered for the Seven Standards the triceps dip requires the use of multiple muscles across multiple joints to give a thorough workout.

The Triceps Dip is a functional exercise disguised in plain sight; from pushing yourself out of a comfy chair to lifting yourself through the loft hatch. Everyday activities are usually performed once as you transition into another activity or movement but imagine if you were an older adult and suddenly found yourself unable to push out of a deep chair. Or worse, unable to push up from the floor after a fall. These situations are often the result of a gradual decline in muscle strength and joint function, possibly due to prolonged disuse. This need not be the case with movement repetition, when a physical activity becomes a structured exercise that can improve strength and function. And if this can happen in older adults (which research overwhelmingly supports!) then it can certainly happen at any age before then.

Be warned, our third body weight Standard is tough when performed correctly. We therefore offer a range of preparatory exercises that may turn out to be your end goal. But that is fine with us and it may be more than fine for you. If for example you are an older adult reading this book (one of many we hope) then mastering the first two preparatory exercises may be the difference between getting yourself off the floor and not getting yourself off the floor after a trip or fall.

For those looking for a different challenge the triceps dip may be a new movement for you to preform and perhaps one you haven't seen before. It requires strength, a degree of shoulder flexibility, and balance in your upper body. There may be a process of motor learning that is required – your brain making new connections in order to perform a new movement. And this learning can be done in the comfort of your own home using the backs of dining chairs, outdoors on playground structures, and even on scaffolding trestles (seen with our own eyes!). Wherever you learn to perform a proper triceps dip you will get the same results – strength, control, and respect from fellow body weight athletes.

Read on to see how the triceps dip develops much more than the triceps muscles.

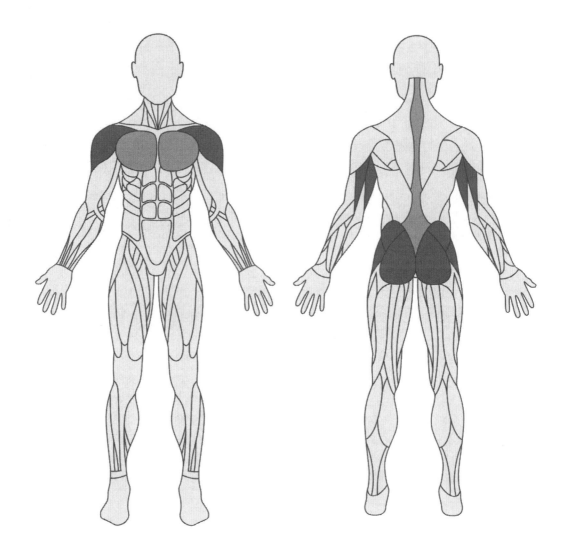

FIGURE 3.1: The Anatomy of the Triceps Dip: Triceps, deltoid, pectoralis major, erector spinae, and gluteus maximus muscles.

The triceps muscle is situated on the back of each upper arm, creating the shape or definition to the straightened arm as it hangs by your side. This is shown in Figure 3.1.

It is a three-headed muscle, from which it derives its name, with three fleshy parts that taper together to form a single tendon at the back of the elbow. When the triceps muscle contracts against resistance it pulls the elbow joint straight (extension), like when pushing yourself up from a deep chair.

The triceps muscle takes its origins from two key locations. The important thing to know here is that one head crosses up over the back of the shoulder joint.

This means that the triceps also pull on the shoulder joint to draw it backwards. If you've ever performed a 'triceps kick-back' type of exercise in the gym then you will have worked the triceps muscle over both the shoulder and elbow joints.

As the body is lowered during the dip the shoulder joint moves backwards (extension) but this is due to the action of the front shoulder muscles lowering the body in to position. These shoulder muscles, the anterior deltoids (shown in Figure 3.1), then contract and shorten to move the shoulder back to the start position. Depending on the body angle during the dip the 'pecs' (pectoralis major) might also get a workout.

If the technique is performed as outlined in the next section then much of the body weight stays back over the shoulders and elbows rather than coming forward over the chest. This requires good control and support through the trunk and pelvis, with the body angled at about 30 degrees to the vertical.

Like all good body weight exercises, especially those collated in this book, the triceps dip activates multiple muscles throughout the body to give you an all-over workout. To keep the body inclined by about 30 degrees the extension muscles of the spine and hips are recruited. These muscle hold tension to keep the spine and hips fixed whilst the upper body executes the dip. These muscles; the erector spinae and gluteus maximus, can be seen in Figure 3.1.

Key Features Of The Triceps Dip

Like the other Standard exercises, the triceps dip has various key features that are unique. Keep these features in mind when performing Standard Three: the triceps dip.

• Arms should be straight and elbows locked in the start position
• Elbows should bend to 90 degrees (preferably more) on each rep
• Head and neck should remain neutral and comfortable throughout
• The effort should come from the upper body
• The legs should not swing to create momentum
• A pause at the top and bottom of the exercise should take place

Performing The Triceps Dip

Now that you have covered a little anatomy and are aware of the key features of the triceps dip, you are ready to learn how this exercise is performed.

Where To Do It

You will need access to some dip bars (or a suitable replacement) for the triceps dip. The stand alone version is ideal for a full, unassisted dip.

How To Do It

1. Grab the dip bars with both hands, palms facing inwards.

2. Straighten your elbows and allow your legs to hang beneath you. Your torso should be vertical and your head and neck should be in a neutral position.

3. Bend your elbows and begin to lower yourself towards the ground. Allow your elbows to flare out at whatever angle is comfortable.

4. Continue lowering yourself, allowing your upper-body to tilt forwards if needed.

5. Aim to get your elbows to at least 90 degrees, preferably a little more.

6. Pause for a second at the bottom position.

7. Push up through your hands and arms and keep going until your elbows are straight and your torso returns to a near-vertical position. This counts as one repetition.

Teaching Points

The triceps dip can be as challenging as the pull-up for some, requiring a combination of strength, good mobility at the shoulders, and balance in your upper-body. Therefore, if you find it tough do not worry - see the preparatory exercises next that will help you in your aspirations to achieve this Standard. To achieve this technique fully you should concentrate on the balance of the body through the arms and the ability to reach 90 degrees bend at the elbow at the lowest part of the exercise.

When To Progress

The aim with the triceps dip is to perform 5 reps without stopping, with the elbows reaching 90 degrees on each rep. Once you can do this you will have mastered another one of the Seven Standards!

To help you master this Standard we have gathered together a set of preparatory exercises that will help in developing the necessary strength and function. These exercises are presented in the following sections, starting with the "ledge dip with bent knees".

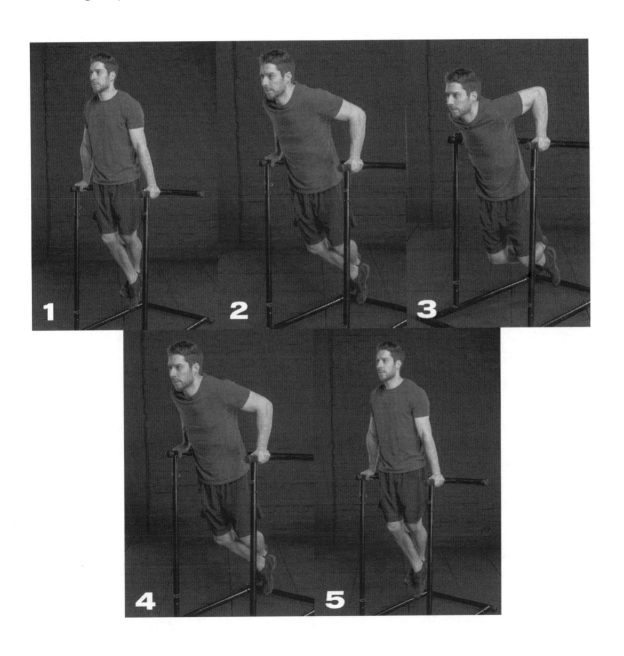

Ledge Dip With Bent Legs

The first stage of learning the triceps dip is the ledge dip with knees bent. A ledge dip is much easier than the full triceps dip, but still uses many of the same muscle groups. Using a ledge and having bent knees is the easiest version, and will allow complete beginners to access the exercise.

Where To Do It

You will need some floor space and a platform of some kind. You can use an exercise step, a stair, or even the edge of a chair or sofa, as long as the platform is strong and stable. You can even use a windowsill or a kitchen worktop, as long as it is stable and safe. Your hands should be shoulder-width apart. Try a height of around 30–45cm or so for the platform.

How To Do It

1. To perform the ledge dip, place your hands behind you on an exercise box, bench, step or raised platform, with your fingers facing forwards.

2. Stretch your legs out in front of you, keeping your knees slightly bent and planting your feet flat on the ground. Keep your back close to your hands and the surface on which they rest.

3. Bend your elbows and start to descend, until your elbows are bent at a 90-degree angle, if possible. You may be limited here by your shoulder flexibility; if this is the case, just descend as far as your mobility allows.

4. Pause for a second, and then push up to return to the start position. This counts as one repetition. Repeat.

Teaching Points

If you struggle with the ledge dip use your legs to help by bending the knees more and stepping your feet back slightly. Push up through your legs. This will take some of the weight off of your arms.

When To Progress

Move on to the next stage when you can do 10 reps with your elbows reaching at least 90 degrees, whilst performing the exercise with bent knees.

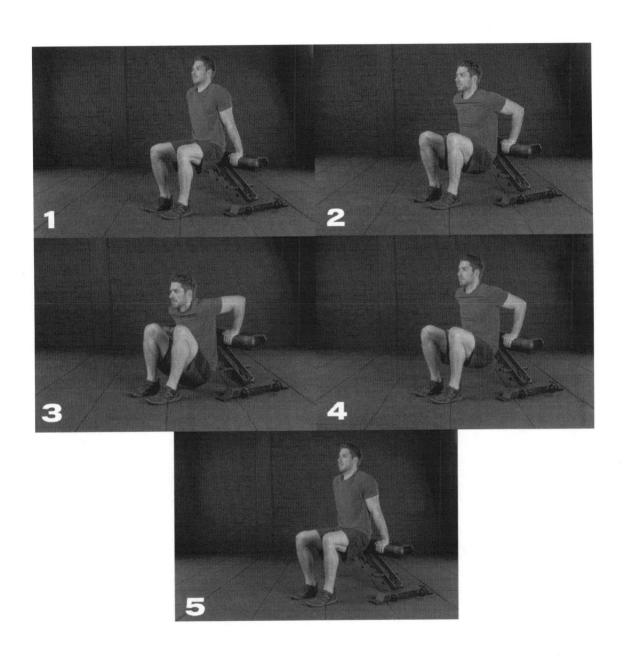

Ledge Dip With Straight Legs

Once you are proficient with the ledge dip with bent legs (Preparatory exercise 3.1), you can straighten the knees to make it more difficult by moving more weight on to your arms.

Where To Do It

Use the same platform that you used for the ledge dip with bent knees, but make sure you have the extra room in front of you to stretch out your legs.

How To Do It

1. To perform the ledge dip, place your hands behind you on an exercise box, bench, step or raised platform, with your fingers facing forwards.

2. Stretch your legs out and straighten your knees, balancing on your heels. Keep your back close to your hands and the surface on which they rest.

3. Bend your elbows and start to descend, until your elbows are bent at a 90-degree angle, if possible. You may be limited here by your shoulder flexibility; if this is the case, just descend as far as your flexibility allows.

4. Pause for a second, and then push up to return to the start position. This counts as one repetition.

Teaching Points

If you find that having straight legs is too difficult then add a very small bend in the knees by bringing your feet in towards you. Keep doing this until you can perform the exercise properly. As you progress and get stronger, move your feet back out to straighten your knees. If this is too easy then place a step of some kind under your feet. This will place more body weight back on to the arms.

When To Progress

Move on to the next stage when you can do 10 reps with your elbows reaching 90-degrees on each rep, with straight knees.

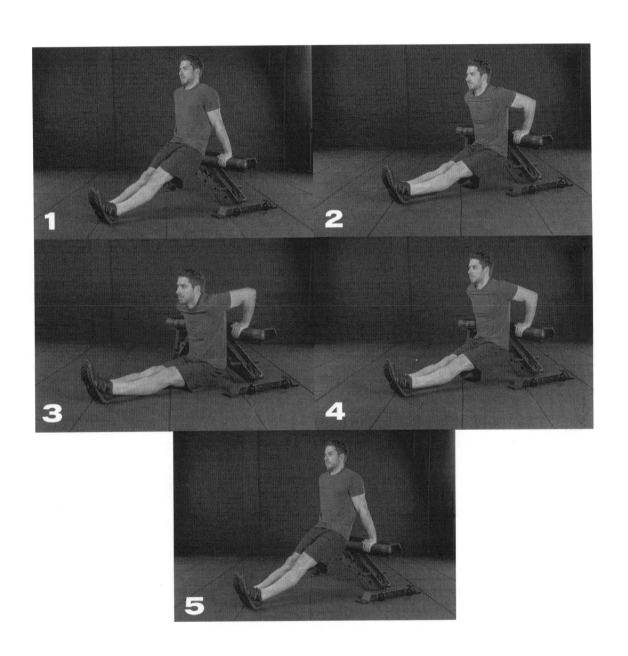

Kneeling Triceps Push-up

We are now going to look at a variation of the push-up. You may be thinking; *why are they including a push-up exercise in the triceps dip section?* Well, it is all to do with strengthening the triceps, which are the pushing muscles of the arms. Preparatory exercise 3.3, the kneeling triceps push-up, is ideal for building strength in the triceps, taking you one step closer to Standard Three - The Triceps Dip!

Where To Do It

You will need some floor space, and an exercise mat or padded surface to cushion your knees. A folded towel works well under the knees.

How To Do It

1. Kneel down and place your hands on the floor, hands shoulder width apart.

2. Stretch your knees out behind you until your shoulders, hips, and knees form a straight line, and your arms are almost vertical from floor to shoulder.

3. Bend your elbows but, and this is the important part, keep your upper arms and elbows tucked in tight to your sides!

4. As you lower yourself towards the floor allow your elbows to move backwards, so that your arms graze your torso. This will make your triceps work extra hard.

5. Keep going until your chest reaches the ground, or as far as your strength allows. Then push up to the start position again, keeping your elbows tucked in to your sides. This counts as one rep.

Teaching Points

The hardest thing about the kneeling triceps push-up is that your chest muscles cannot help much. The larger 'pec' muscles are made redundant by keeping those elbows tucked in! This puts all of the resistance onto the backs of your arms - the smaller triceps muscles. If you struggle, try using a raised platform as you did for the earlier stages of the push-up, and then reduce the height of the platform as you get stronger. Alternatively, perform a shallower triceps push-up through a smaller range of motion.

When To Progress

Move onto the next stage when you can do the kneeling triceps push-up for 5 reps without stopping, managing to get your chest to the floor each time.

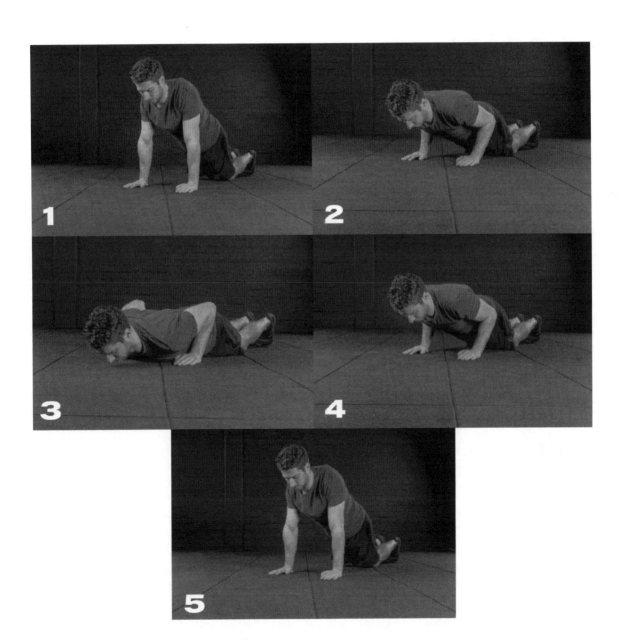

Shallow Triceps Dip

We are now going to move onto the dip bars for real! Congratulations on making it this far as it takes real strength. The shallow triceps dip will get you used to the movement pattern of the full triceps dip, but with a reduced range of motion. This is great for building specific strength and movement familiarity for Standard Three - The triceps dip.

Where To Do It

You will need access to a set of dip bars, or something else suitable for dips. The backs of two chairs will work great, as will other similar objects. Please ensure they are solid and secure. Some outdoor spaces like parks now have dedicated exercise equipment that may include bars suitable for the triceps dip.

How To Do It

1. Place both of your hands on the bars, palms down and fingers pointing away from you.

2. Push yourself up so that your arms become straight at the elbow. Allow your legs to relax below you, or if the floor is too close, cross your ankles and bend your knees to avoid them hitting the floor.

3. Bend your elbows and begin to lower yourself down, but only a small amount! Perhaps 30 - 45 degrees of elbow bend.

4. Lower yourself as far as you are comfortable, pause for a second, and then push yourself back up again. This counts as one repetition.

Teaching Points

If you struggle to hold yourself up on just your arms and find that supporting your entire body weight is a good workout, then practice holding the top position of the triceps dip until your upper body gets stronger. As you become stronger you will be able to lower yourself down further over time.

When To Progress

Move on to the next stage when you can do 5 reps with at least a 45 degree bend in the elbow, and your feet are off the ground throughout.

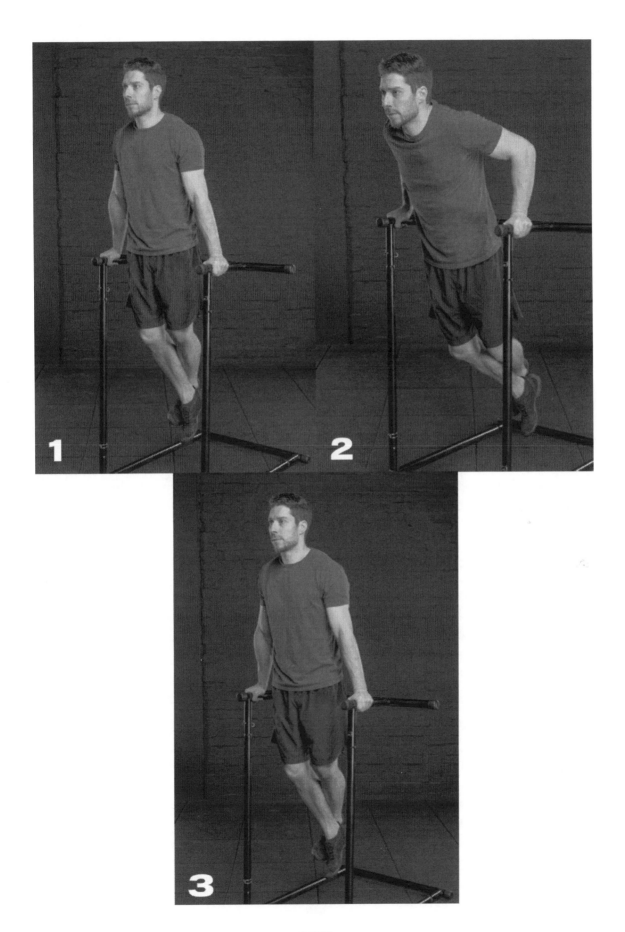

Negative Triceps Dip

This exercise is a great progression from preparatory exercise 3.4. The negative triceps dip is included here to build greater strength. You may recognise the use of 'negative exercises' in the other Standards. This process is also essential in learning a controlled technique for the full triceps dip.

Where To Do It

You will need access to a set of dip bars, or something that allows you to perform dips safely and securely, like the backs of two solid chairs, or other apparatus. See Preparatory exercise 3.4 for more advice on this.

How To Do It

1. Grab the dip bars with your palms facing downwards and your fingers pointing away from you.

2. Push yourself up until your arms are straight at the elbow. This is the top position. Allow your legs to relax, or if the floor is too low, cross your ankles and bend your knees.

3. Bend your elbows and begin to lower yourself down as slowly as possible. Keep lots of tension in the upper body and exert maximum force! Lower yourself as far as possible until you can support yourself through your arms no longer.

4. As soon as you get to the bottom of the position, place your feet on the ground and rest. This counts as one repetition. Now return to the start position.

Teaching Points

The key with this exercise is to do it slowly and keep control of the movement! At first you may struggle to perform these slowly, but as you get stronger you will be able to lower yourself under complete control. In no time you will reach your goal.

When To Progress

Move on to the next stage when you can perform a negative triceps dip that takes you 20 seconds from top to bottom.

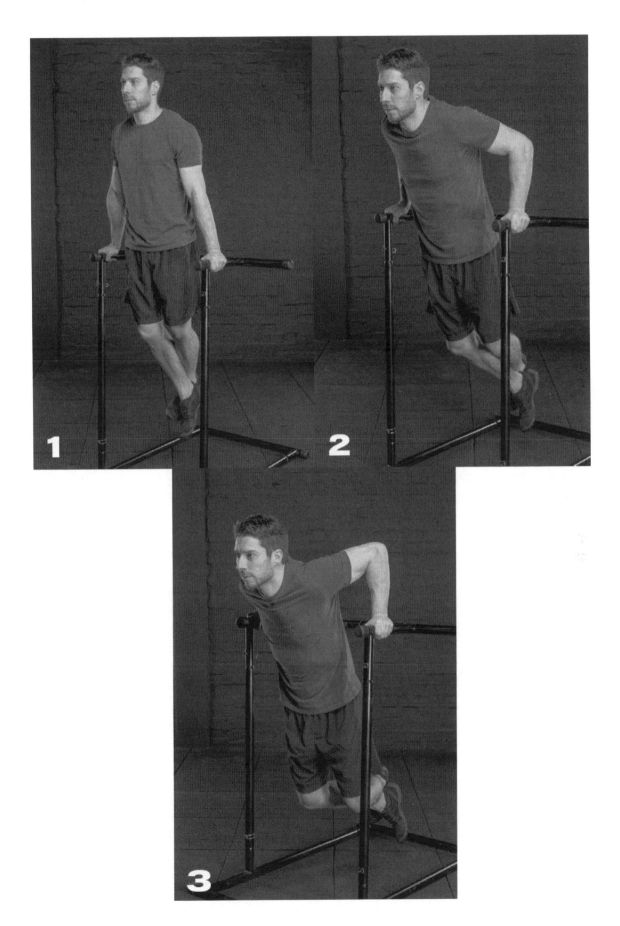

Assisted Triceps Dip

As valuable as the negative triceps dip is (preparatory exercise 3.5), working with a full range of motion version is needed for training the muscles and movement patterns for Standard Three - The triceps dip.

Where To Do It

You will need an assisted dip machine for this exercise. These can be found in many gyms, and are often paired with pull-up bars to create a pull-up/triceps dip station.

Alternatively you can work with a partner who can provide some support by cupping under your bent knees to offload some body weight. A further option for assistance is to purchase some elastic therapy band and tie a length between the bars to create a sling that you can cradle your knees in. These bands comes in different strengths (and colours) and so can provide variable amounts of support. Please ensure you tie the knot tightly if using this equipment and that the band is free of tears or defects.

How To Do It

1. To perform the assisted triceps dip, set the weight on the machine for at least 75% of your own body weight. For example, if you weigh 80 kilograms (175 pounds) you should have at least 60 kilograms (130 pounds) on the machine. If using the alternative methods of assistance (suggested above) then there will be a degree of guesswork based on your perceived effort level.

2. Grab the bars with your palms facing downwards and your fingers pointing away from you. Rest your knees or feet on the support pad, your partner, or therapy elastic sling.

3. Bend your elbows and begin to lower yourself down. Keep going until your elbows are at 90 degrees, or until you reach the limit of your flexibility.

4. Pause for a second, and then push yourself back up again. This counts as one repetition.

Teaching Points

The beauty of the assisted triceps dip is that the difficulty can be adjusted incrementally (if using the assisted machine), so that you can progress gradually as needed. You can also progress or modify the depth of each assisted dip.

When To Progress

Move on to the final stage - Standard Three: The Tricep Dip - when you can perform 5 reps with 25% of your body weight on the machine. For example, if you weigh 80 kilograms (180 pounds), then you would need 20 kilograms (45 pounds) on the machine. If using our alternative methods of assistance then you should feel like you are doing 75% of the lifting and your partner or therapy band is taking only 25% of your load.

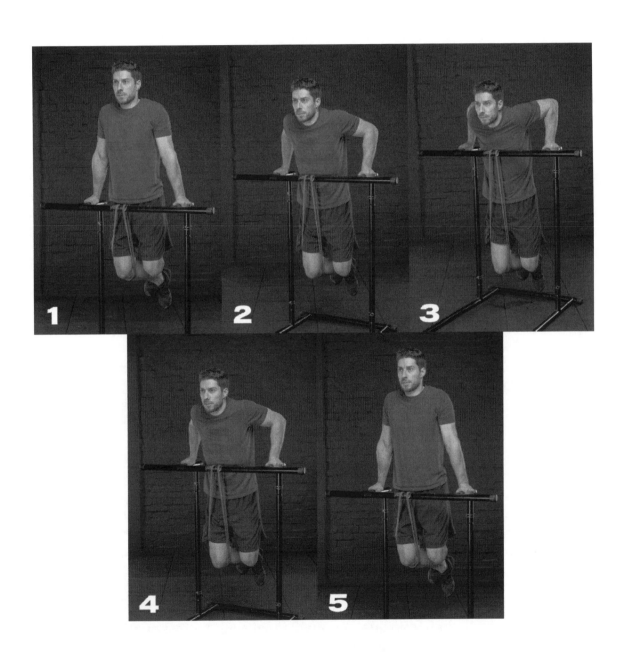

10.4 Standard Four: The Squat

Of the Seven Standards chosen for this book the squat is perhaps the most important of all. To perform the full (deep) squat, even without additional load, there is a requirement for a large range-of-motion and strength at the hip, knee, and ankle.

The squat is a movement that children seem able to perform effortlessly during play but gradually with age this ability seems to be lost. Why is this? The literature reports that between 10% and 20% of adults in developed countries like the UK, United States of America, and Australia have osteoarthritis of the knee. On the whole this condition appears to be more prevalent with age from the mid-thirties through to eighty years plus. It can be associated with pain and a lack of range-of-motion at the joint.

Another way to look at these trends is to consider the time passed since early age. For example, someone in their mid-thirties may not have completed a deep squat for 15 years, while an individual in their mid-seventies may not have completed a regular deep squat for fifty years! There are many factors involved in the development of osteoarthritis of the knees and hips but a joint not receiving regular mobilisation and distribution of its lubricating fluid is likely to stiffen with time. Such a state may be a factor in the later development of osteoarthritic changes in the knee and hip.

So, back to the squat. When was the last time you completed one? A deep squat that brings your buttocks right down towards your heels?

Don't jump up and try it just now. When you start working towards this Standard go easy and get a feel for what your hips, knees and ankles are currently capable of. Achieving the squat is the end-goal of this Standard so please do not try to do too much too soon.

In addition to developing and maintaining range-of-motion in the lower limb joints the squat also prevents age-related muscle loss, known as sarcopenia. This degenerative muscle loss, especially around the lower limbs, has been implicated in increasing frailty and risk of falls in later life. But the reasons for squatting are apparent for all ages – a toned rear, increased muscle mass in the thighs, improved jumping power in sports. If nothing else it will make getting off the sofa that little bit easier! Have we made the case yet for Standard Four: The Squat?

Before we focus on the technique of squatting let's outline the anatomy involved in the greatest of body weight exercises.

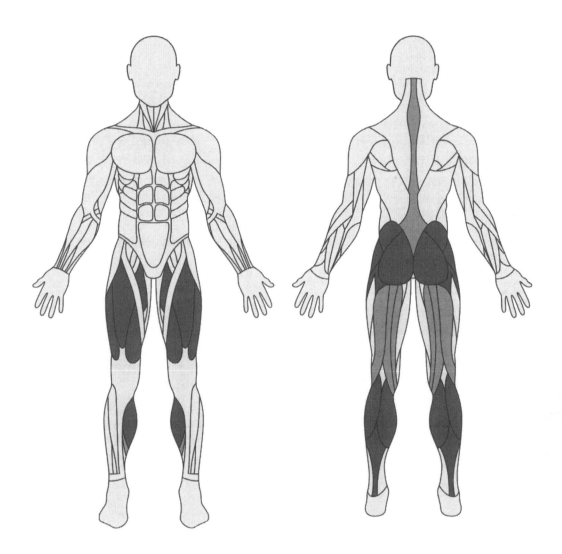

FIGURE 4.1: The Anatomy of the Squat: Gluteus maximus, hamstrings, quadriceps, erector spinae, gastrocnemius and soleus.

As discussed above, the squat is mainly used to focus on the range-of-motion and strength in the lower limbs. Specifically the joints of the hips, knees, and ankles; but as always we'll introduce you to a few 'hidden extras' along the way. That's the beauty of body weight exercise!

During the squat the hips flex (bend) to allow the trunk to come forward and maintain weight over the feet. The further into the squat you move the more flexion is needed at the hips. All the while, one of the largest and most powerful muscles in the human body – the gluteus maximus, is lengthening to lower the body towards the ground. Once the hips have reached their lowest point in the squat the gluteus maximus muscle begins to contract whilst shortening, driving the hips back towards the start position.

Assisting the gluteus maximus muscles in driving up the hips is the hamstring muscle group. All three muscles of the hamstring group cross the back of the hip joint and contribute weakly to hip joint extension. The hamstrings are situated on the back of the thigh and can be seen in Figure 4.1.

While the hamstring muscles sit round the back of the thigh their counterpart, the quadriceps muscle group, sit on the front of the thigh. Here the four quadriceps muscles contract to create straightening (extension) of the knee. From the lowest position of the squat this bulk of muscle pulls at the knee to lever the body upwards. To lower the body back to the squat position the quadriceps will lengthen under tension. In order to maximise both phases of the muscle contraction it is beneficial to maintain a steady controlled rhythm of movement throughout. This will also help to keep your balance over the feet. Figure 4.1 shows the location of the quadriceps muscle group.

As with all body weight exercises, and especially those making the Seven Standards, there are wider demands on the body that give a fuller workout. The squat is certainly no exception. During both the up and down phases of the squat there are muscles supporting and controlling the movements at the ankle. At the lowest point of the squat the ankle is said to be in dorsiflexion. This movement may be limited by some stiffness in the ankle or tightness in the muscles at the back of the lower leg. Build up slowly! From this position the muscles at the back of the lower leg contract as the body is forced upwards. These muscles, the gastrocnemius and soleus, give the calf its characteristic appearance. They can be seen in Figure 4.1.

Finally, to maintain an upright trunk posture we must also consider the role of the spinal extensor muscles, especially those of the lumbar (lower) spine. When the trunk flexes forwards it is these muscles that prevent you falling forwards. On the return movement the spinal erector muscles shorten to restore a straight lumbar spine. The demands on the trunk are increased if the squat is performed under additional load such as a barbell across the shoulders. Figure 4.1 shows the location of the spinal extensor (erector spinae) muscles.

Key Features of the Squat

Some key features of the squat are as follows:

• Feet shoulder width apart, knees tracking toes
• Descend to where the thighs are horizontal
• The lower back should remain straight
• The hips should move back and down during the technique

• A pause should happen at the bottom position of the exercise
• The head and neck should be held in a neutral position

Performing The Squat

Now that you have learned the unique aspects of the squat and why it forms an important part of a balanced body weight exercise routine, you are ready to learn how to perform the squat .

Where To Do It

You will need some floor space, with room enough for you to squat down and move your arms forward. You can also use a chair or platform behind you for safety.

How To Do It

1. Stand with your feet shoulder width apart, toes pointing out slightly.

2. Your arms should be hanging loosely by your sides, head looking forward in a neutral position.

3. Bend your knees and position your hips backwards as you do so.

4. Allow your arms to rise up as you descend, to help with balance.

5. Continue bending your knees, with the hips moving back and down.

6. Descend until your thighs are horizontal, or preferably until your hips move below the level of your knees.

7. Hold the end position for a second, and then return to the standing position. This counts as one repetition.

Teaching Points

The squat requires balance and some of this will come from the arms as you lower the body. As your bottom moves backwards reach forwards with your arms for counter-balance. As the knees bend do not allow them to move forwards over the toes as this can add stress to the knees and ankles. The squat is a tricky exercise to master but one that is well worth it. Use the preparatory exercises that follow to help you develop the ability to execute the squat perfectly.

When To Progress

You will have mastered Standard Four: The squat, when you can perform 15 reps without stopping, with your thighs reaching at least a horizontal position and maintaining your balance throughout.

To help you master this Standard we have gathered together a set of preparatory exercises that will help in developing the necessary strength and function. These exercises are presented in the following sections, starting with the sit-stand.

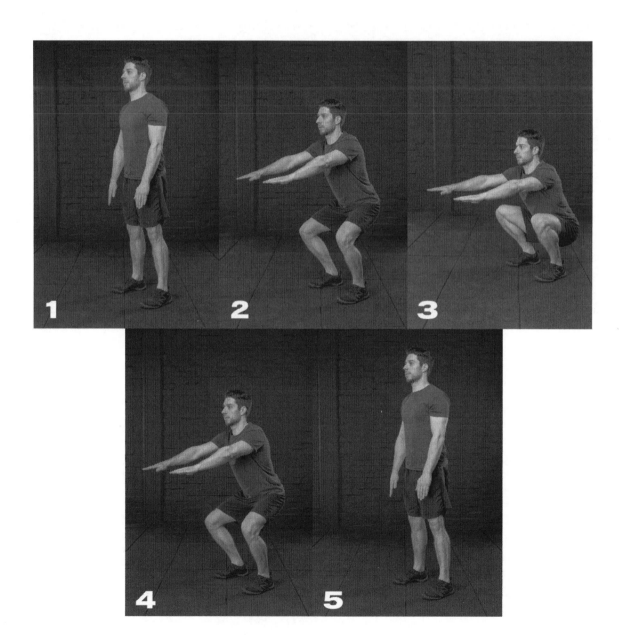

Sit-stand

The first stage in learning to squat is simply sitting down and standing up, preferably using a chair or platform that allows your thighs to be horizontal when sitting. We call this preparatory exercise the sit-stand, and it will familiarize your lower body with the motion and the muscles needed for the squat. This is a very useful exercise for those rehabilitating a hip or knee injury, and also for older adults wanting to improve their lower body strength.

Where To Do It

You will need a stable chair or platform of some kind that is at knee height. Ideally it should allow you to sit down so that your thighs are in a horizontal position.

How To Do It

1. Stand in front of your chair or platform, with the backs of your legs just touching the object.

2. Your feet should be approximately shoulder apart, toes pointing out slightly. Your arms should be by your sides.

3. Now bend your knees and position your hips backwards. Sit down slowly under control, moving your arms out in front of you to help balance.

4. Sit down fully, moving your torso back until you are sitting upright. Pause for a second, and then reverse the movement so that you stand up again. On the return phase lean forward slightly to initiate the pelvis / hip roll. This counts as one repetition.

Teaching Points

If you have trouble standing up without using any momentum, then use your arms to help you. You can push down on the sides of the chair or platform, or swing your arms up to give you some momentum. As you get stronger you can reduce the amount of help that you give yourself from your upper body.

When To Progress

Move on to the next stage when you can do 15 reps without stopping, and without pushing up with your arms.

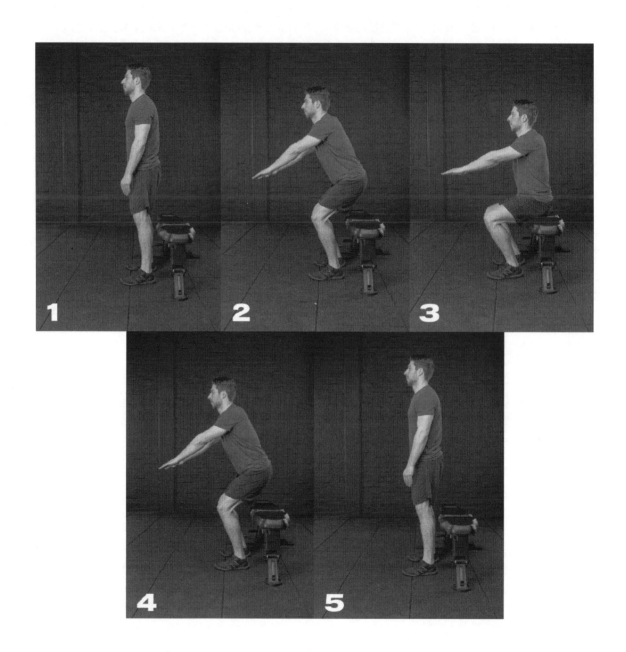

Shallow Squat

Once you have gotten to grips with the sit-stand (preparatory exercise 4.1), you can remove the chair and start performing shallow squats, with or without a support. Shallow squats are exactly what they sound like; squats where you only squat down a little way. This ensures you don't overstress your leg muscles, and that you can safely return to a standing position from the squat position.

Where To Do It

You will need some floor space, and if you prefer, you can do this with a chair behind, to catch you if you cannot stand back up again. You may benefit from a countertop or windowsill in front of you to place your hands on for steadiness.

How To Do It

1. Stand with your feet approximately shoulder width apart, with your toes pointing out slightly.

2. Make sure that you are standing up straight, with your eyes looking ahead and your head and neck in a neutral position.

3. Bend your knees and position your hips backwards, squatting down slowly. Only bend your knees a small amount though!

4. Keep squatting until you feel tension on the muscles at the front of your thigh, pause for a second, and then stand up again. This counts as one rep.

Teaching Points

Shallow squats should be achievable for most people, as you are in control of the depth of the squat. If you are a beginner, or don't have much confidence, just bend your knees very slightly at first, so that you know you can stand back up again. As your confidence and strength increases squat down a little lower each time.

When To Progress

Move on to the next stage when you can do 15 reps with your thighs reaching 45 degrees, with no use of support in front of you.

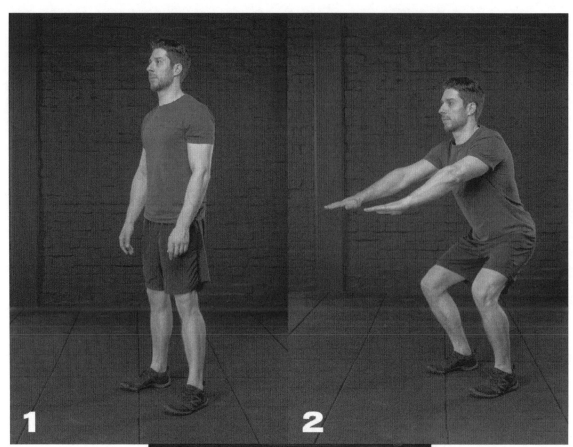

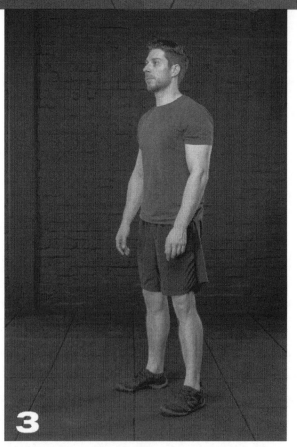

Shallow One Leg Squat

You might be thinking that a one leg squat sounds very difficult! But don't worry, this exercise is actually easier than it sounds. By putting the emphasis on one leg, the shallow single leg squat allows you to develop each hip, knee and ankle. This is important for developing equal contribution from both legs and for improving balance around the ankles.

Where To Do It

You will need some floor space, and also a chair or platform behind you for safety. This way, if you descend too low and cannot get back up, you can simply drop onto the chair and rest. You may benefit from a countertop or windowsill in front of you to place your hands on for steadiness.

How To Do It

1. Stand on one leg, with the other lifted off the floor a small amount. Raise your arms to aid in your balance.

2. Keeping your head and neck in a neutral position, bend your knee and start to squat down. Do not allow your knee to push forward of your foot position. Only bend your knee a small amount to begin with! Focus on your balance and technique rather than depth of squat.

3. Descend as far as you can before you feel strain on your thigh, keeping your free foot from touching the ground.

4. Reverse the movement and stand back upright again. Go slowly and maintain your control and balance. This counts as one repetition. Be sure to work both legs equally!

Teaching Points

This exercise might seem a little difficult at first because of the balance element. Remember that you can control the range of motion directly so that the emphasis is on balance and technique. When starting, only bend your knee a very small amount. As you get stronger increase the range of motion as much as you are comfortable with. As you improve you can also reduce any external support for balance.

When To Progress

Move onto the next stage when you can do 10 reps on each leg, with up to about 45 degrees of bend in the knee and no external support for your balance.

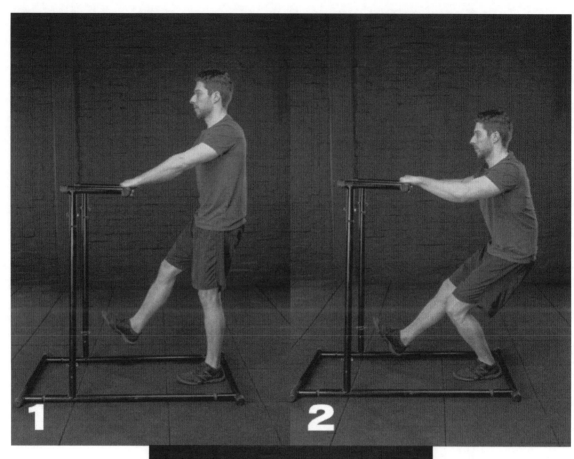

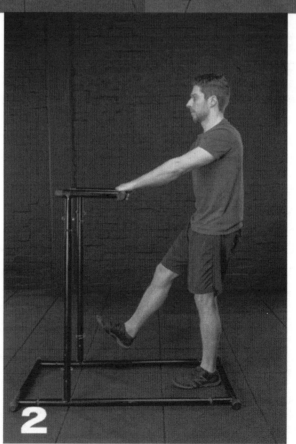

Crouch

Where preparatory exercise 4.3 developed a shallow range of movement at the hips, knees and ankles, the Crouch takes you through a fuller range. Crouching down is difficult for many people to do, often because they have had no need to do it for several years and so have lost the ability. It can however be used as a starting place for developing a proper squat.

Where To Do It

You will need some floor space to perform this exercise. You may also want to use a mat if you would like to protect your knees. A folded towel works well for this also.

How To Do It

1. Stand with your feet shoulder width apart, with your toes pointing out slightly.

2. Make sure that you are standing up straight, with your eyes looking ahead and your head and neck in a neutral position.

3. Bend your knees and position your hips backwards, squatting down slowly. Lean forward slightly and have your hands ready to touch the ground.

4. Keep squatting until your hands reach the ground, and gradually move into a crouched position. Your knees should be bent, heels up, and hands on the floor.

5. There are two options now:

– you can hold this position to stretch out the hips, knees, and ankles. We recommend a few seconds to 30 seconds depending on comfort.

– you can push up to return to the standing position. This is one rep.

Teaching Points

The crouch may challenge you at first depending on your low back, hip, knee and ankle mobility. The best way to improve joint stiffness is to gradually and gently work in to that stiffness. Keep practicing this exercise but if you find you have joints that are particularly stiff or painful then please seek an assessment from a qualified health or medical professional. Having a healthy musculoskeletal system requires mobility and strength!

When To Progress

You should move onto the next stage when you can perform the crouch for 30 seconds with no problems, or when you can do 5 reps getting into and out of the crouch position. Even better, when you can do both of these.

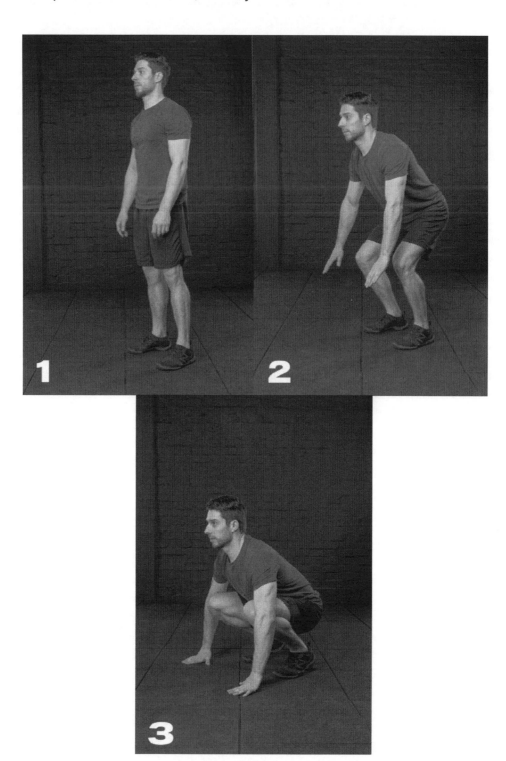

Assisted Squat

As with many of the other preparatory exercises in Body weight Basics, you can use an assisted version of the exercise to help get the body familiar with the movement. The assisted version of the squat can be very helpful, especially if you are still building your flexibility but want to increase your strength.

Where To Do It

There are a number of places where you can do assisted squats. One way is to use a door frame. You can hold onto the door frame with your hands and squat down, using your arms to guide you and pull you up if needed. If you have access to a gym then you may be able to use suspension training equipment, which are handles on long cords. Such equipment is very popular and can even be found in many home-gyms.

How To Do It

1. Firmly grab the equipment you are using (be that a suspension trainer, door frame, or other solid object) and stand with your feet shoulder width apart, toes pointing out slightly.

2. Make sure that you are standing up straight, with your eyes looking ahead and your head and neck in a neutral position.

3. Bend your knees and position your hips backwards, squatting down slowly. Keep hold of the equipment with your hands, controlling the descent with your legs and arms.

4. Squat down as far as you can, pause for a second, and then stand up, using your arms as needed to help pull up. When you reach the standing position this is one repetition.

Teaching Points

The great thing about the assisted squat is that you can alter the amount of assistance that you give yourself at every stage of the exercise. If the top portion is easy then you only need give yourself a little assistance, and at the bottom (where it is more difficult) you can give yourself more help. Pay attention to how much your arms are helping, and try to reduce the amount of assistance as you progress and get stronger.

When To Progress

Move onto the next stage when you can perform 10 reps whilst only giving yourself a little help. This would ideally be about 25% of the overall effort, meaning your legs are pushing the remaining 75% effort. This may be difficult to judge, so come back to this stage if you feel the next exercise (4.6) is too difficult for you.

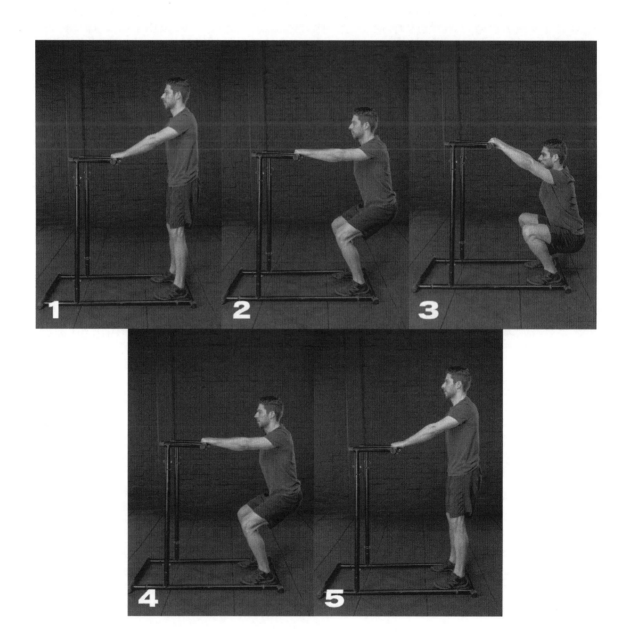

Deep Squat Position

In order to get the most out of the squat it is ideal if you can squat down low. This maintains or improves the function of your joints and also works the muscles through their full length. To do this you can practice holding a deep squat position. This will stretch and mobilise the muscles, ligaments, and capsules around joints for a deeper squat.

Where To Do It

You will need some floor space to perform this exercise.

How To Do It

1. To perform the deep squat position, place your feet flat on the floor, heels shoulder-width apart and your toes pointing slightly out.

2. Stretch your arms out in front of you and keep your eyes looking forwards, head and neck neutral.

3. Bend your knees, position your hips backwards and squat down as far as you can. Keep your lower back as straight as possible. Keep your heels on the ground with the feet firmly planted for stability.

4. The position you are trying to achieve can be seen in image 4.6. If you cannot get down this low, go as low as you can. Hold for 30 seconds, or as long as you are able to. You can then either stand back up (if you can), or move out of the squat position and then stand up from a crouch.

Teaching Points

To open up the hips you can press your elbows into the insides of your knees and push outwards. This will stretch the hips and allow you to get deeper into the squat. This is a particular favourite of one of the authors!

When To Progress

Move onto the next stage when you can comfortably hold the deep squat position for at least 30 seconds. Ideally you want your lower back to be straight, and your hips open with the feet flat and stable on the ground. This can take some time to get right, so keep practicing. It will be well worth it!

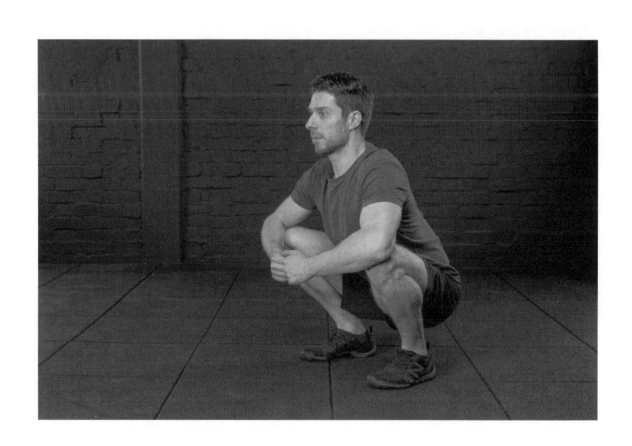

10.5 Standard Five: The Lunge

In the previous Standard we praised the merits of the squat. We may have even gone as far as to say it was the ultimate lower body workout. We stand by that – the squat is an awesome body weight exercise, but if you want to add an extra dimension to your leg workout then you need the lunge! The added benefits of the lunge could be summed up in two words (this could be a short section!) – Balance and control.

The squat is static from the perspective of its base of support, whereas the lunge requires a shift in foot position. It becomes dynamic in comparison and also switches-up the muscle activity, and so unlike any of the other Standards in this book it makes successive repetitions different to the last (assuming you do as we later suggest and alternate legs!).

The lunge requires a step-standing posture meaning that one foot is ahead of the other. Depending on your technique, your base of support could therefore be narrow and less stable. This challenges your balance and causes your brain to light up as it hurriedly coordinates incoming and outgoing signals to maintain your body over your feet.

As a result of the muscle activity maintaining balance, it is not unusual to feel an ache around the ankle after a lunge workout. If this is something you experience then it may suggest you are developing something called proprioception – the ability to sense body position and the amount of effort required to maintain that position.

If you are a 'mature' reader of this book then performing regular lunges in a safe and controlled environment may reduce your risk of trips and falls.

If you are a younger reader of this book then it may also reduce your risk of trips and falls. The lunge does not discriminate based on age!

In addition to challenging standing balance the lunge varies from the squat in that it creates a trailing leg. The angles created at the hip, knee and ankle in the trailing leg are quite unlike any other exercise (body weight or otherwise). Muscles and joints are therefore stretched and strained through different ranges and patterns. The major benefit to this is the variation of stress on the exercising body, meaning that repetitive strain injuries are less likely. It may also add to the resilience of the body in unpredictable sports like soccer or tennis where joints can be stressed in unusual positions. Regular lunge training could therefore reduce injury risk in these instances. Although the squat in Standard Four might be our overall favourite for the legs the lunge comes a very close second with its added extras!

The Anatomy of the Lunge

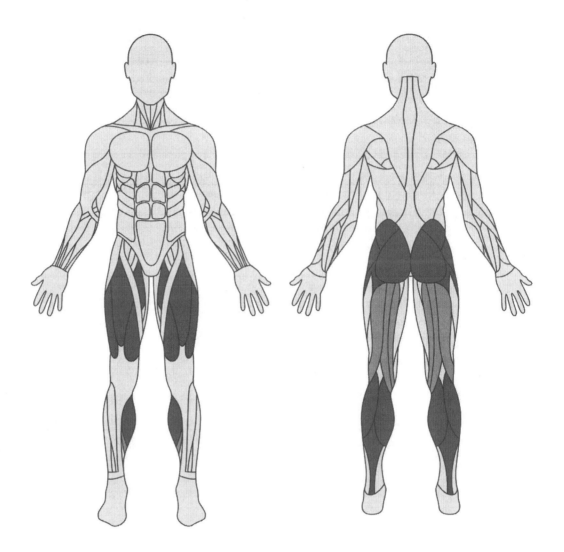

FIGURE 5.1: The Anatomy of the Lunge: Gluteus maximus, hamstrings, quadriceps, gastrocnemius and soleus.

Many of the muscles and joints worked during the lunge were also the focus of the squat in the previous Standard, however, the mechanics of the lunge give a whole different workout to these muscles. The asymmetric nature of Standard Five: The Lunge means that focus is placed on muscles unilaterally. As we talk through the anatomy of the lunge we will assume that we are stepping with the left foot forward, but to even-out the effect then the reverse will be true for a forward right foot.

A forward left foot creates hip flexion (bending) on the left, which is increased as the body lowers into the lunge position. The left knee begins in some degree of extension (straightening) as the left foot steps forward but gradually lowers into flexion by the end of the lunge. For both of these movements there is muscle lengthening under tension, predominantly at the left gluteus maximus (buttocks) and the left quadriceps muscle group. These muscles are illustrated in Figure 5.1. At the hip there may also be some weak assistance from the hamstrings muscle group.

Some research has suggested that eccentric muscle contractions, where the muscle lengthens under tension, can lead to greater muscle mass compared to concentric (muscle shortening) contractions. This increase in muscle mass is normally measured as muscle girth. Eccentric muscle contractions are also thought to cause greater increases in strength, but you should bear in mind that this increased strength will most likely be specific to the types of movement being trained.

Whilst the hip and knee of the leading leg (left leg in this example) are moving into flexion under load, the left ankle is moving into increasing dorsiflexion (when the shin moves closer to the top of the foot – or vice versa). As this is also happening under tension the powerful gastrocnemius muscle at the back of the lower leg is also contracting eccentrically. The gastrocnemius, or calf muscle, is shown in Figure 5.1. The lunge will therefore give a great workout for the muscles of the lower leg and ankle.

While all of the above is happening on the leading leg the trailing leg is having a completely different challenge. The right hip is extended (straightened) throughout the lunge whilst the right knee moves into flexion. This creates a different stress on the quadriceps (Figure 5.1) compared with the leading leg, not least because part of the quadriceps muscle spans both the hip and knee. The quadriceps of the trailing leg contract eccentrically but do so whilst under a greater stretch. In the trailing leg the ankle remains at a fairly fixed angle.

So far we have seen mostly eccentric contraction of the major muscles shown in Figure 5.1. As the lunge reaches the lowest point there is a momentary hold whereby the muscles discussed hold their length before shortening as the body returns to the start position. As the body drives upwards against gravity the quadriceps and gluteus maximus muscles contract forcefully as they shorten. The force developed by these muscles needs to be rapid to create momentum in the upward movement.

All of the movements described here require a good functional ROM at the hips, knees and ankles, as well as balance and coordination. When progressed slowly the lunge will also develop joint range of movement as well as strength and stability in the muscles around joints. It really is an exercise worth adding to your workout routine.

Key Features of the Lunge

Some key features of the lunge are as follows:

• Step distance should be larger than normal walking gait
• The torso should remain upright throughout the exercise
• Both knees should reach at least 90 degrees of bend
• A pause should be performed at the end of the movement
• The heel should hit the ground first when stepping forward
• The head and neck should remain neutral, eyes looking forward

Performing the Lunge

Now you have covered the anatomy of the lunge and the key features of Standard Five, it is time to learn how to effectively perform the lunge.

Where To Do It

You will need some floor space for this exercise, and if you perform the stepping-forward version of the lunge, plenty of room in front of you. This will be dictated by the number of reps and your step length but we recommend five to seven metres.

How To Do It

1. Stand with both feet shoulder width apart, arms relaxed by your sides.

2. Take a large step forward with your right foot, slightly larger than your normal walking gait.

3. As your right foot hits the floor start to bend both knees so that you sink towards the ground. The body movement should be downwards rather than forwards.

4. Continue bending your knees and descend towards the ground. Your torso should remain upright.

5. Pause when both knees are an inch or two from the ground. Now push through both feet, and as you come up return your rear leg towards the standing position. This counts as one repetition.

Teaching Points

As with the other lunge exercises that form the preparatory exercises for this Standard (see next), make sure that you practice with both feet in the forward position. This way you will ensure that your individual leg strength develops equally.

When To Progress

You will have mastered this Standard when you can perform 8 reps without stopping, with both legs in the forward position, and maintaining your balance throughout.

To help you master the the lunge we have gathered together a set of preparatory exercises that will help in developing the necessary strength and function. These exercises are presented in the following sections, starting with the step-stand.

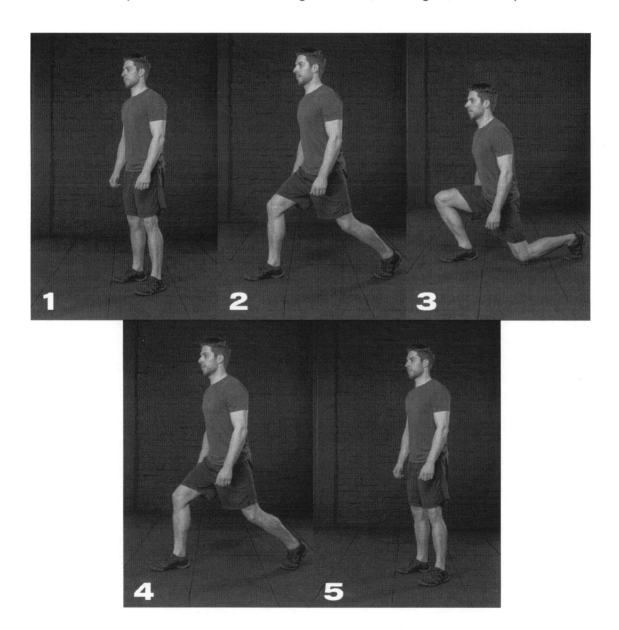

Step Stand

The first stage in achieving the lunge is the step stand. This is useful for those who are a little unsteady on their feet, and for those unfamiliar with the lunge technique.

Where To Do It

You will need some floor space for this exercise.

How To Do It

1. Stand with your feet shoulder width apart, toes pointing out slightly, and your arms relaxed by your sides.

2. Now lift one foot off the floor and take a large step forward that is slightly longer than your usual walking gait.

3. As your front foot touches the ground bend both knees very slightly.

4. Pause for a second, and then push off hard with your rear leg and bring it forward to meet your front foot, so that you arrive back in the standing position again. This counts as one repetition.

Teaching Points

The step stand is a basic component of the lunge but it is fundamental to appreciating the balance, distance and feel of the lunge step. If you feel comfortable you can bend your knees a little more to do a mini lunge, but don't go too far at this stage. Also, make sure to step forward with alternate legs each time, so right foot forward, left foot forward, right foot forward, and so on. If you want to challenge your balance and are in a safe environment then once in step standing you can try closing your eyes whilst maintaining your balance.

When To Progress

Move on to the next stage when you can do 8 reps on each leg without stopping or losing your balance. You may get to this stage very quickly, in which case you are ready for the next preparatory exercise (5.2)

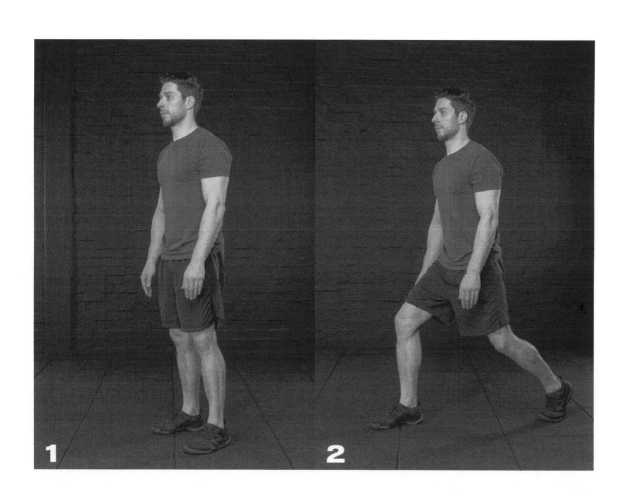

Hip Flexor Stretch

The hip flexors consist of a few muscles at the front of your hip that when relaxed allow the hip to extend. Increasing your flexibility here can make the lunge more comfortable to perform. Good mobility here also allows your torso to stay upright with one leg forward and one leg backward.

Where To Do It

You will need some floor space and an exercise mat for your knees.

How To Do It

1. To perform the hip flexor stretch, place your right foot and your left knee on the floor.

2. Move your front foot forward until your leading hip and knee are at right-angles. Ensure your rear knee is under your trunk and that you are aiming for an angle of 90 degrees or more in the rear knee.

3. Lean forward and shift your weight towards the leading knee, letting your target hip open up. You should feel a stretch in the top of your rear leg. Keep your torso upright as much as possible.

4. Hold this position for 30 seconds, then change legs and repeat.

Teaching Points

If you progress well with the hip flexor stretch, you can make it more difficult by moving the leading foot and rear knee further apart. This increases the intensity of the stretch. Try also raising the arm on the target hip side in the air as this will ensure there is no leaning of the trunk.

When To Progress

Move onto the next stage when you can get into the stretch position easily without feeling too much of a stretch. The sensation should be comparable on both sides. It really is up to you how far you take this exercise, as you can continue to increase your flexibility with continued training. This exercise is great for niggling hip and low back pain. For further detail on this we refer you to our other book - *Bulletproof Bodies: Body weight Exercise for Injury Prevention and Rehabilitation*.

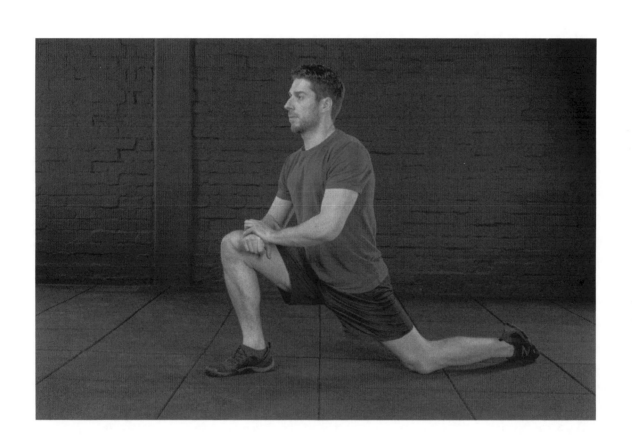

Lateral Lunge

The lateral lunge is a mix of the lunge and the squat exercises. It is not a lunge per se, but uses many of the same muscles, and helps to improve balance. It can also be used as an effective exercise in its own right, to improve your strength, mobility and balance in the lower limbs.

Where To Do It

You will need some floor space, and room to move sideways for at least ten feet or so (if available).

How To Do It

1. Stand with your feet shoulder width apart, arms by your sides.

2. Lift your left foot off the ground, and step left about 12 inches or so.

3. Now bend both knees and squat down as low as you comfortably can (practice with the squat exercises if you need to - see section 9.4)

4. Stand up and move your right foot towards your left until you arrive in the standing position. This counts as one repetition.

Teaching Points

If you are struggling to perform the lateral lunge then try only squatting a small distance, and only moving the feet a little way left and right. This will make the exercise easier to control. As you progress you can step further and squat lower each time.

When To Progress

Move on to the next stage when you can perform ten reps to the left and right without stopping or losing your balance, with your knees reaching at least 45 degrees when squatting.

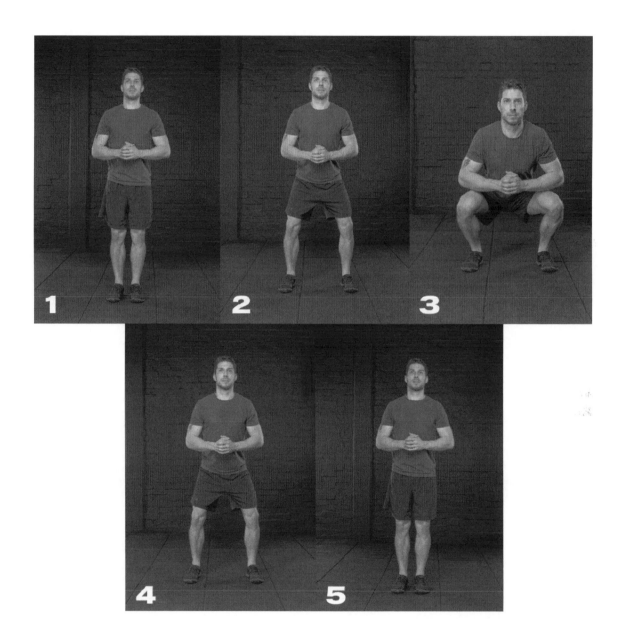

Shallow Lunge

Like many of the other exercises we have given in Body weight Basics, the shallow version of the full lunge allows you to approximate the full exercise but with a reduced range of motion. This will make the exercise easier and more accessible, but still allows for gains in strength, mobility and balance.

Where To Do It

You will need some floor space for this exercise.

How To Do It

1. Stand with your feet shoulder width apart, arms relaxed by your sides.

2. Step forward with one of your feet by a distance of about two feet.

3. As your front foot touches the ground your front knee will pass forward toward your lead foot while your rear knee will descend towards the floor. Control yourself into a lunge position, but only lunge to a small depth.

4. Pause for a second, and then do either of two things:

– Push off hard with your front foot, and return to the standing position. You can now step forward with the opposite foot for another rep.

– Push off hard with your rear foot and step forward, returning to the standing position. You can now step forward with the opposite foot for another rep. For this version you will effectively be walking forwards and so will require more space to complete consecutive repetitions.

Teaching Points

With the shallow lunge you use a reduced range of motion and so can control the difficulty by controlling the depth of the lunge. As you progress with this preparatory exercise you can increase the depth of the lunge, building strength and mobility as you go.

When To Progress

Move onto the next stage when you can perform 8 reps on each leg with your leading knee getting to at least 45 degrees of flexion. Maintain your standing balance throughout.

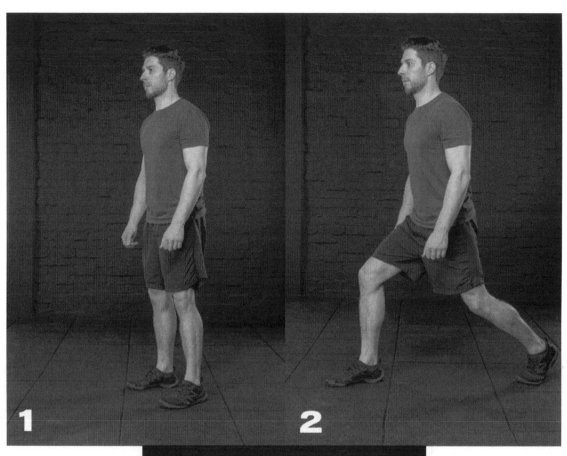

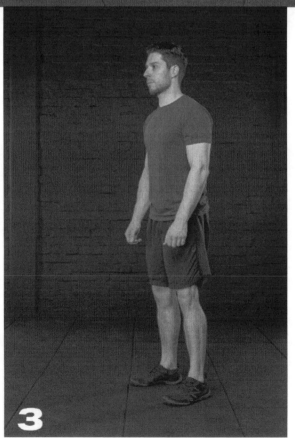

Lunge Balance

Keeping your balance can always be a challenge when completing a good-quality lunge, especially when in the bottom position. To develop this, and to build up some strength and control in the legs, you can do the lunge balance.

Where To Do It

You will need some floor space to perform this exercise.

How To Do It

1. Stand with your feet shoulder width apart, arms relaxed by your sides.

2. Step forward with one foot for a distance of least two feet.

3. As your front foot touches the ground your front knee will pass forward toward your lead foot, while your rear knee will descend towards the floor. Control yourself into a lunge position aiming to get both knees to 90 degree angles.

4. Hold this position for 30 seconds. Raise your arms out by your sides to aid balance.

5. Once you have held the bottom position for the required amount of time, step forward or backward out of the lunge. Then rest, and repeat with the opposite foot forward.

Teaching Points

The lunge balance can be made easier by reducing the range of motion. Simply bend your knees a small amount to make the exercise easier. You can also decrease and increase the distance between your feet to adjust the difficulty. To make the exercise easier decrease the distance, and to make it more difficult increase the distance. The lunge balance can also be regressed or progressed by altering the amount of time held in the balance position.

When To Progress

Move onto the next stage when you can hold the position for 30 seconds comfortably and without losing balance, with both knees held at 90 degrees.

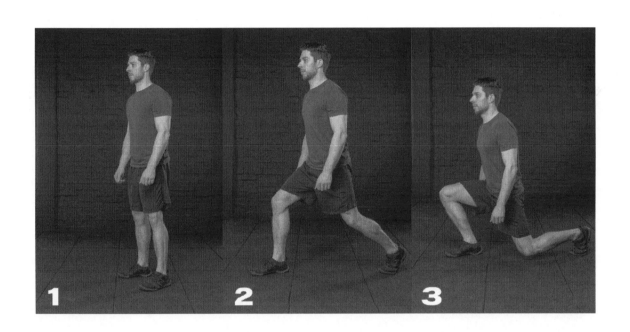

Static Lunge

We now come to the static lunge, which uses the same body position as the normal lunge, but instead of returning to the standing position each time, you will keep both feet where they are and perform reps. This is the part referred to as "static". This places a greater demand on the leg muscles, developing more strength.

Where To Do It

You will need some floor space for this exercise.

How To Do It

1. Stand with your feet shoulder width apart, arms relaxed by your sides.

2. Step forward with one foot by a distance of at least two feet, or slightly more than your usual walking gait.

3. Bend both knees slightly as your front foot touches the ground. This is the starting position for the static lunge.

4. Now bend both knees at the same time, and lower yourself towards the ground, until your knees are at 90 degrees or as low as you as you can comfortably get. Keep your torso upright.

5. Pause for a second, and then push up to the starting position. Do not step back to the standing position but instead remain in step-standing. This counts as one repetition.

Teaching Points

You can use a reduced range of motion to make the static lunge easier. To make it more challenging you can also increase the range of motion. Work both sides of the body equally, performing equal numbers of reps with your right foot forward and your left foot forward.

When To Progress

Move on to the next stage when you can perform 8 reps without stopping, with your knees reaching 90 degrees each time. Make sure you can do this with both legs in the forward position.

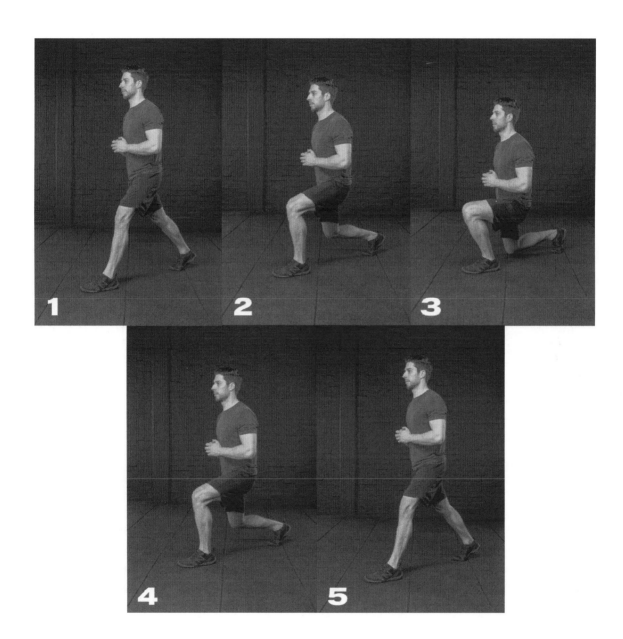

10.6 Standard Six: The Plank

The plank is like no other exercise in this book. Its requirements are quite unique and the rewards can be far reaching. From posture, to the push-up, to the planche; the ability to hold a perfect plank can improve performance in all of these.

In the Standards covered so far we have identified a common theme – movement. If you flick through the body weight exercise Standards One to Five you will see that there are phases of movement from muscles lengthening and shortening under tension. We have described these muscle contractions as eccentric and concentric phases respectively.

In the plank you will notice an absence of movement. Once in position it is a static hold. That's right, no movement required. All you have to do is hold the position, and if you can do this for a minimum of 90 seconds with good form then you have achieved our sixth Standard of body weight exercise. Sounds easy, right?

When muscles are held in equal length under tension, maintaining the position of joints, this is termed an isometric contraction. During the plank there will be resistance to this fixed position in the form of gravity. Pulling down through the shoulders, spine, trunk, pelvis and legs gravity will eventually cause those static muscles to shake, shudder, and then give-out. The lower back will start to sag and the pelvis will roll forwards. The thighs will begin to burn as your knees sink towards the ground. Resisting this strain can be easily done, but doing so while holding good alignment is much more difficult, and this is where the concept of posture comes in.

Posture comes in all different shapes, with some being much better than others. From a 'front to back' perspective there is a degree of alignment through the head, spine and pelvis that is considered more ideal. It involves holding the natural curves of the spine and 'tucking' the tummy. It requires good tone in the gluteal (butt) muscles and stability around the shoulder blades. All these requirements are amplified in the perfect plank, and so by training in this Standard it is possible to increase bodily awareness and control for an 'ideal' posture.

The hold position required for the plank approximates that of the push-up, as seen in Standard Two of this book. Training the plank will therefore improve control and muscular endurance of the trunk during the push-up.

And if you wish to continue your adventure in body weight exercise, these attributes will better prepare you for more advanced exercises like the legendary planche. What more could you ask from one exercise?

The Anatomy Of The Plank

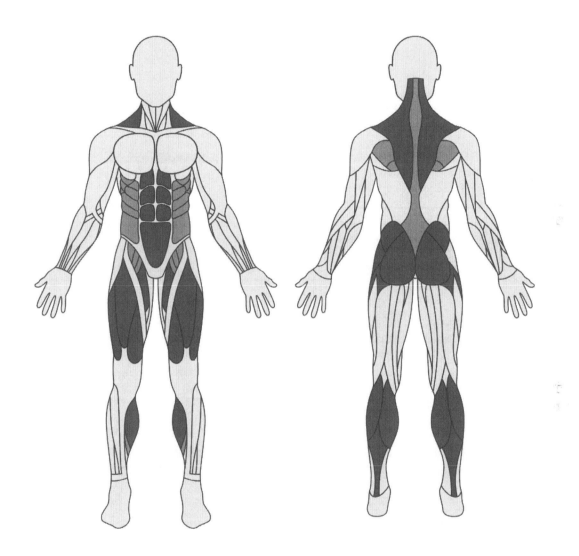

FIGURE 6.1: The Anatomy of the Plank: Erector spinae, rectus abdominis, transverse abdominus, hip flexors, and external abdominal oblique. Also, trapezius, rhomboids, rotator cuff, serratus anterior, gluteus maximus, quadriceps, soleus and gastrocnemius.

The plank is often referred to as a "core" exercise meaning that it predominantly targets the muscles of the spine and trunk. This is true. You only need to try the exercise once (with proper technique) to find out where it strains the most. But like all body weight exercises the plank also requires the efforts of multiple muscles throughout the body. We shall review the target muscles briefly in this section.

Core muscles, as referred to in most workouts, are the muscles around the spine and abdomen that have a key role in creating stability. They are often deeper muscles that provide the body with improved function rather than aesthetics. So while you may not get the ultimate "six-pack" abdomen from doing the plank you may find that you have improved posture, a tighter or flatter looking tummy, or even a reduction in your low back pain. The deeper stabilisation muscles found at the "core" include the transversus abdominus and rectus abdominus at the front of the abdominal wall. These muscles are shown in Figure 6.1.

When doing the plank some scientific literature has also reported increased muscle activity in the erector spinae muscles and the external abdominal oblique muscles. The erector spinae muscles run along the spinal column and, as the name suggests, act to keep the spine straightened (erect). They can be seen in Figure 6.1.

The external oblique muscle of the abdomen is the largest of three flat muscles covering the front and side of the abdominal wall. This muscle helps to compress the abdominal cavity, keeping the tummy flat. In a world of poor posture, activating this muscle may be the quickest fix for a protruding abdomen! Contraction of the external oblique muscles increase the pressure in the abdominal cavity and in turn may raise blood pressure. If you have any concerns about your general health then we recommend an assessment from a health or medical professional before beginning a new exercise programme. Figure 6.1 shows the external abdominal oblique muscles.

The aim of the plank is stability, support and control. These attributes are developed in the trapezius, rhomboids, and serratus anterior of the upper body to support the position of the upper spine and shoulder blade (scapula), as shown in Figure 6.1. The deep shoulder muscles of the rotator cuff have also been implicated in the plank to control the shoulder joint during load-bearing through the arms.

Muscles around the hips, knees and ankles are also activated in the plank to hold the position. At the hips the gluteus maximus muscles help to hold the pelvis and hip joints in best alignment, while the quadriceps work at both the hip (in part) and knee during the plank. Finally, the gastrocnemius and soleus muscles at the back of the lower leg contract isometrically to hold the weight of the legs over the balls of the feet. These muscles are shown in Figure 6.1.

Key Features of The Plank

Some key features of the plank are as follows:

• The elbows should be positioned underneath the shoulders
• The forearms should remain flat against the floor throughout
• The head and neck should remain in a neutral position
• The hips must sit in line with the shoulders and ankles
• The lower back should stay tight and straight
• The spine should stay neutral throughout

Performing the Plank

Now you know the anatomy and key features of the plank it is time to learn how to perform the perfect technique.

Where To Do It

You will need some floor space and an exercise mat or something to cushion your elbows.

How To Do It

1. Place your forearms on the ground, with your shoulders resting directly over your elbows.

2. Stretch your legs out behind you with your knees and toes on the ground.

3. From here raise your hips into the air and lift your knees off the ground.

4. Straighten your legs and ensure your shoulders, hips, knees, and ankles are in a straight line.

5. Keep your head and neck in a neutral position, and hold this position for the required amount of time.

Teaching Points

When performing the plank it is important to maintain the height of the hips and not let them drop out of alignment with the shoulders and knees. This can strain the lower back and reduce the effectiveness of the core muscles, making it harder to hold the position. It is essential to not hold your breath during this exercise, but instead try to breathe in to the bases of the lungs.

When To Progress

The aim with this Body weight Basics Standard is to hold the plank position for 30 seconds without stopping or losing the ideal position. Once you can do this you will have mastered another one of the Seven Standards!

To help you master the plank we have gathered together a set of preparatory exercises that will help in developing the necessary strength and function. These exercises are presented in the following sections, starting with the prone pelvic tilt.

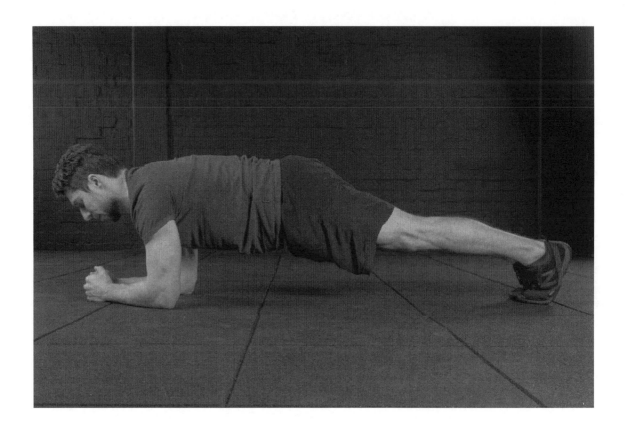

Prone Pelvic Tilt

When learning the perfect plank it is important to learn how to hold a neutral spine posture and to engage the core muscles. The prone pelvic tilt can be used for this.

Where To Do It

You will need some floor space, enough for you to lie down without restriction. You may like to do this exercise on some carpet, a mat, or other soft and dust-free surface.

How To Do It

1. Lie face down, with your arms crossed in front of you and your forehead resting gently on your hands.

2. Gently press your pelvis into the ground by engaging your core muscles and tilting your pelvis. It may feel like your low-back is flattening out.

3. Focus on the pelvic tilt and you may feel your pubic bone press in to the floor / mat. This should feel like the opposite of arching your low-back.

4. Hold the position for 10 seconds, and then rest.

Teaching Points

Trying to engage the core muscles can feel strange at first. A tip is to gently rock the pelvis backwards and forwards; arching and flattening your low-back. When activating the deep abdominal and pelvic muscles it can sometimes feel a bit like when you try to stop yourself urinating mid-flow.

When To Progress

Move onto the next stage once you can engage the muscles necessary to control the tilt in the pelvis. You should be able to do this with ease, feeling relaxed and not holding your breath.

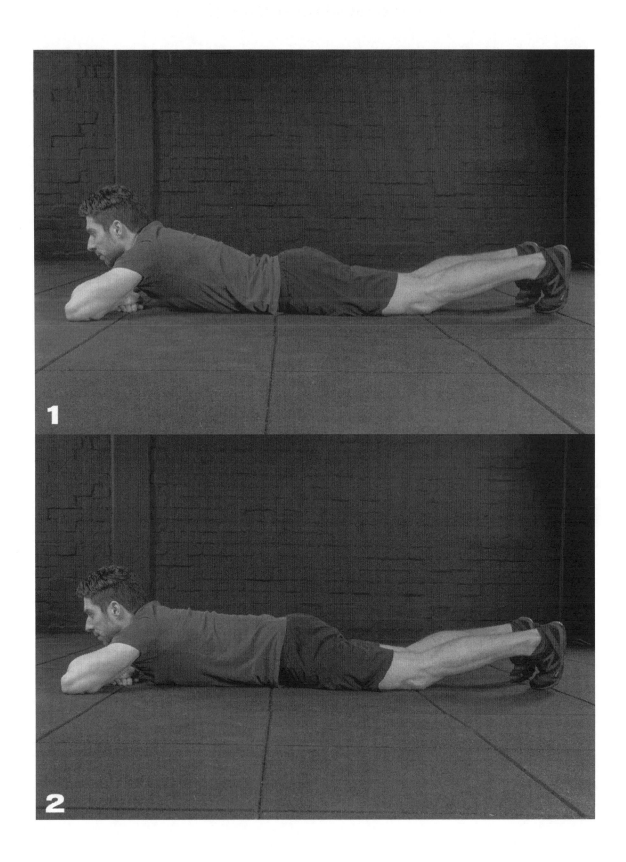

Platform Push-up Hold

The second stage in developing the plank is the platform push-up hold. If you have worked through the preparatory exercises for Standard One: The Push-up, then you may already be at an advantage here.

Where To Do It

You will need a raised platform, the same as you used when performing the push-up (Standard One). This can be a set of stairs, an exercise box or step, the edge of a sofa or bed, or anything else that is sturdy and at the height of your knees when standing. If you have something that can be adjusted in height this will allow you to vary the difficulty of the exercise.

How To Do It

1. Place your hands on the platform, shoulder width apart, with your fingers splayed slightly. Maintain straight arms.

2. Stretch your feet out behind you and balance on your toes.

3. Make sure that your body is aligned, and hold this position for as long as possible. Aim for 10 to 20 seconds initially.

Teaching Points

The hardest part is keeping the body aligned throughout the hold, and not letting the hips drop or the spine sag due to gravity. If you struggle to hold the position for long (10 to 20 seconds), take a break by moving one foot forward and resting for a second, and then move this foot back into position and carry on.

When To Progress

Move onto the next stage when you can hold the position for 30 seconds without resting and without too much effort required to hold the alignment.

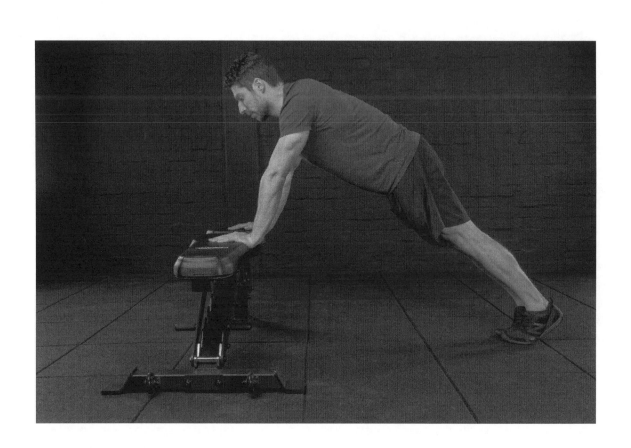

Bridge

The bridge is not an 'abs' exercise, but instead develops multiple core and pelvic muscles. You may think that the core is only made up of the muscles in the front of the trunk, but we can also include the muscles of the lower back. The muscles of the hips and buttocks will also assist with pelvic control and therefore may improve posture and spine health.

This version of the bridge is a more accessible version than the full version (which is featured in our book - *Bulletproof Bodies: Body weight Exercise for Injury Prevention and Rehabilitation*).

Where To Do It

You will need some floor space, and a mat to lie down on.

How To Do It

1. Lie down on your back, with your arms relaxed by your sides.

2. Plant the soles of your feet on the ground and pull your feet in towards your bum, so that your knees move beyond 90-degrees of flexion.

3. Squeeze your glutes and brace your core muscles and raise your hips from the ground. Keep the back of your head in contact with the ground, with your neck relaxed and not under strain. Keep your arms relaxed by your sides.

4. Keep raising your hips until your shoulders, hips, and knees form a straight line. Hold this position for as long as possible, aiming for 10 to 20 seconds initially.

Teaching Points

At first you may find it difficult to raise your hips up to the required level. It helps to concentrate on tensing your glutes, or buttock muscles. This will help engage the correct muscles in your core, and help you to get into the right position. If the front of your hips feel tight then try preparatory exercise 5.2: Hip Flexor Stretch.

When To Progress

Move onto the next stage when you can perform the bridge for 30 seconds without resting, and without excessive strain whilst holding the end position.

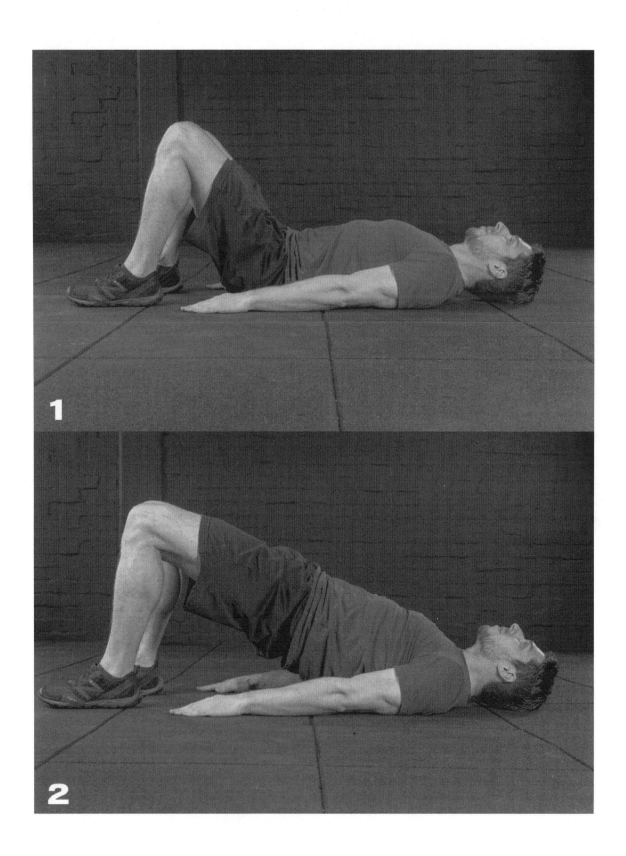

Kneeling Plank

The kneeling plank is a great way to train the plank but with a reduced level of resistance. As the name suggests, the kneeling plank is the same as the full plank, except that the lower body is supported on the knees and not the toes. This reduces the amount of body weight that you are working with, and so makes the exercise easier.

Where To Do It

You will need some floor space, and an exercise mat for your knees and elbows. A folded towel can work well here for comfort.

How To Do It

1. Kneel down and place your forearms on the ground, with your elbows shoulder width apart. Make a lightly-clenched fist with your hands, and tense your upper body to take the strain through your arms.

2. Move your knees backwards until your torso forms a straight line, and your upper arms are vertical.

3. Once you are in this position, hold it for as long as possible, aiming for 10 to 20 seconds initially.

Teaching Points

As this is your first exposure to the plank position, you may find it a little difficult. The key is to keep the hips in line with the shoulders and knees, and to not let them drop down below this line.

When To Progress

Move onto the next stage when you can hold the kneeling plank for 30 seconds with perfect form and without undue stress throughout.

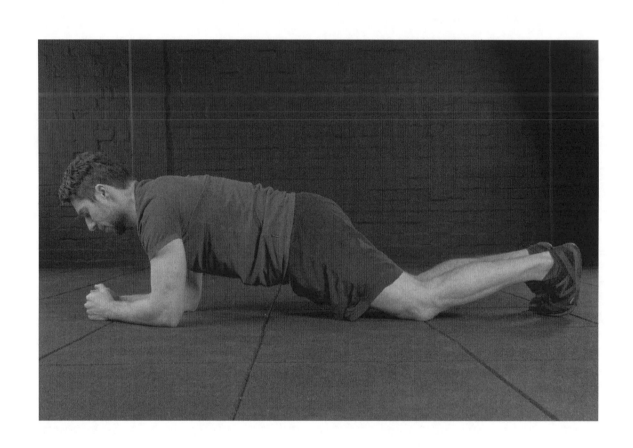

Static Crunch

This preparatory exercise is about developing strength and stamina in the abdominal muscles. The static crunch is the same as the crunch, except that instead of going up and down you will be holding a still position for a set time period.

Where To Do It

You will need some floor space and an exercise mat or cushioned floor.

How To Do It

1. Lie on your back with your arms by your sides and the soles of your feet planted flat on the floor.

2. Draw your feet towards your buttocks until your ankles and feet are comfortable.

3. Now tense your 'abs' and draw your upper rib cage forwards and upwards. This will curl your shoulders off the floor. You are not aiming to "sit up", but curl the top of your spine so that your core develops tension.

4. Keep your head and neck as neutral as possible, and slide your hands along the floor (towards your feet) as you curl up. Avoid excessive bending of your spine and neck as you lift your shoulders from the floor.

5. Once you have curled up as far as you are able, and your shoulders are clear of the floor, hold this position as long as possible, aiming for 10 to 20 seconds initially.

Teaching Points

Some common problems with the static crunch include too much tension in the neck, not enough core strength, and not being able to curl the spine. Keeping the head in a neutral position throughout the exercise can help tension in the neck. Hold your chin out rather than tucking it in and down towards your chest. If your core strength is weak at first then reduce the range of the curl, or aim for a static hold of 5 seconds initially.

When To Progress

Move onto the next stage when you can hold the static crunch for 30 seconds without resting and without excessive strain throughout.

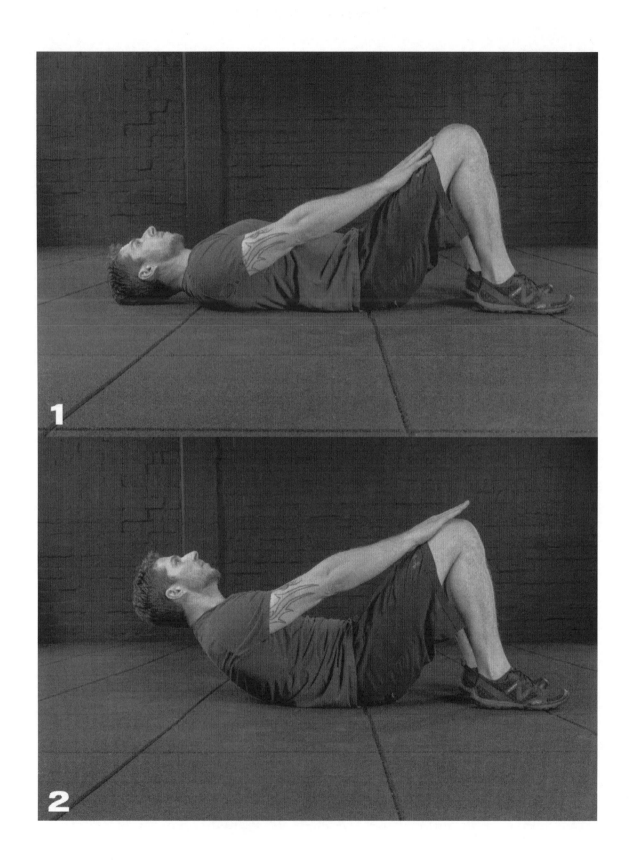

Plank Pulses

The penultimate stage! Plank pulses are a great way to build strength in the plank position, but without you having to hold the position for any length of time. With this preparatory exercise you are required to perform reps instead.

Where To Do It

You will need some floor space and an exercise mat or cushioned floor. A folded towel may be useful to cushion the elbows.

How To Do It

1. Kneel down and place your forearms on the ground, with your elbows shoulder-width apart. Make a lightly-clenched fist with your hands, and tense your upper body to take the strain through your arms.

2. Stretch your legs out behind you and balance on your toes. Raise your hips up so that your shoulders, hips, knees, and feet form a straight line. Hold this position for a second or so, and then lower yourself back down onto your knees.

3. Keep "pulsing" like this, up and down, aiming for 5 to 10 reps.

Teaching Points

Your aim with plank pulses is to spend more and more time in the plank position, and only drop your knees down for a few seconds. Make sure that each time you raise your hips back into the air that you get into the same position. It is easy to let the hips drop and your spine sag as you begin to fatigue. You are much better to hold a good technique (form) for shorter than a sloppy technique for longer.

When To Progress

Move onto the next stage when you can do 30 plank pulses without excessive resting between reps, holding the top position for 2 to 5 seconds each time.

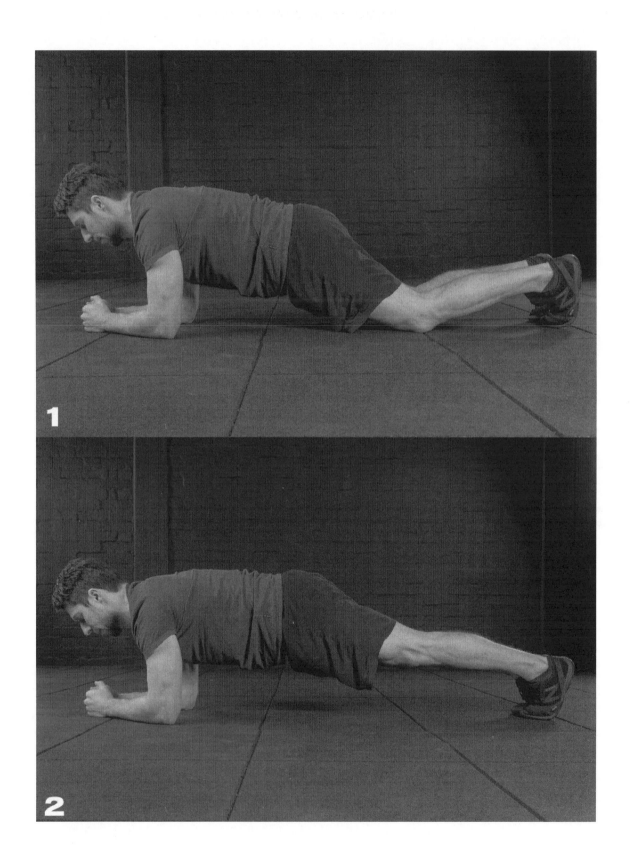

10.7 Standard Seven: Inverted Shoulder Press

The seventh and final Standard of Body weight Basics is an exercise that stands apart from the others. It will turn your world upside-down – literally. As such we issue our disclaimer early for this exercise. Because this Standard involves a head-down position we do not recommend it for anyone with a history of high blood pressure, gastric reflux, or any other condition that you are not sure about. If in doubt we recommend that you seek advice from a suitably qualified health or medical professional.

When pondering over the exercises to include in this book we knew that we wanted to include something for the shoulders. With body weight exercise it becomes a little tricky to load the shoulders in comparison to the gold-standard shoulder exercise that is overhead pressing. There are alternatives such as raising the arms to the side or front of the body, and these can be loaded with body weight, but they just don't cut it.

Our other goal was to maximize the involvement of other body segments, both to reduce workout time and to increase training gains. We feel that the inverted shoulder press ticks all the boxes.

The inverted shoulder press provides an introduction to pressing body weight whilst also developing the body's ability to train in an inverted position. This will help you progress towards body weight calisthenics exercises like headstands, handstands, and German-hangs, if that is your ultimate training goal.

In addition, the inverted shoulder press does something much more important – it develops mobility in the low back and hamstrings (backs of thighs). Tightness in these body areas can be associated with low back pain, and this condition is thought to affect up to 80% of UK adults at some time in their lives.

To assist your development towards completing the seventh Standard we have put together some great preparatory exercises that will challenge your weaknesses and restrictions. Go steady at first and allow your body to adapt. If you stick with it the gains will be well worth it!

The Anatomy of the Inverted Shoulder Press

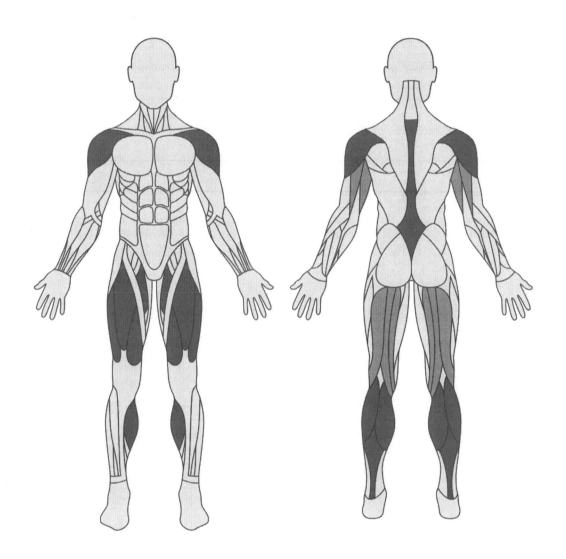

FIGURE 7.1: The Anatomy of the Inverted Shoulder Press: Deltoids, rotator cuff, thoracic spine, triceps, quadriceps, lumbar spine, hamstrings, and gastrocnemius.

The inverted shoulder-press exercise offers a range of benefits to the joints and soft tissues of the body, and these will be outlined here.

The major training impact comes from the position held throughout the inverted shoulder press. For those familiar with yoga you may be reminded of the "downward dog" posture. For those unfamiliar with the downward dog yoga pose we have included this as a preparatory exercise for this Standard. In this pose there is a stretch from fingers to toes. Most noticeable is the stretch felt at the shoulders, middle-spine, hamstrings, and calves.

Whilst holding the start position of the inverted shoulder press there is extension at both shoulders whilst also developing load-bearing stability in the rotator cuff muscles (see Figure 7.1). The thoracic spine is the section of the spinal column sitting between the neck and low back. This spinal region can spend much of its time in flexion due to modern lifestyle postures. In the inverted shoulder press the thoracic spine gets a well-needed extension stretch, easing the strain on muscles, ligaments, joints and intervertebral discs in the area.

Lifestyle postures, such as sitting, can also contribute to shortening in the hamstrings and gastrocnemius muscles (Figure 7.1). There may also be tension in the sciatic nerve and its associated branches that run along the back of the thigh and lower leg. All of these structures are mobilised or stretched in the inverted shoulder press. Go steady at first as straining these structures may cause some irritation if done aggressively.

We've covered some of the anatomy on stretch during our seventh Standard, but we haven't yet revealed the true extent of the strength gains.

The obvious benefit to this exercise is the deltoid muscles (Figure 7.1) that make up the bulk of the shoulders. In the start position the deltoids are holding a static (isometric) contraction. The deltoids then lengthen under tension to move the shoulder joint through adduction to bring the head towards the ground. If you have any concerns about your shoulder strength then we strongly recommend placing a cushion or padded mat beneath your head for this phase. From this position the deltoids contract to push the shoulder joints through abduction. The result is that the head is lifted to the start position.

In addition to the deltoids there is recruitment of the triceps muscles at the back of the upper arms. The triceps muscle (see Figure 7.1) is a three-headed muscle (hence the name) that crosses both the shoulder and elbow joints. In the inverted shoulder press the triceps muscle contracts to straighten the elbow joint during the return phase, and is also responsible for lowering the elbow joints into flexion.

As discussed in previous Standards, eccentric muscle contractions can lead to increased muscle mass when measured as muscle girth and may cause greater increases in strength compared with concentric muscle contractions. These higher gains in strength will be specific to the movement pattern being performed.

Finally, in order to maintain the 'downward dog' posture through the inverted shoulder press the quadriceps muscles of the anterior thighs must maintain a static (isometric) contraction. The action of the quadriceps here is to hold the knees in extension and prevent them buckling.

Now that we have reviewed the extent to which the inverted shoulder press gives a finger-to-toe workout, let's put it into action by examining the ideal technique.

Key Features of The Inverted Shoulder Press

Some key features of the inverted shoulder press are as follows:

• Palms should be pressed flat against the floor
• Legs should be straight, although a small bend in the knee is allowed
• Elbows should bend to at least 90 degrees
• A pause should be performed at the end position
• The spine should remain as straight as possible

Performing the Inverted Shoulder Press

Now that you have covered the anatomy and the key points of the inverted shoulder press you are ready to learn how to effectively perform the final Standard. Due to the "head-down" position, you should not perform this exercise if you have problems with your blood pressure, stomach reflux, or any other medical condition that you are unsure about.

Where To Do It

You will need some floor space to do this exercise, preferably with a non slip surface. You may want to use a mat or similar to cushion the hands.

How To Do It

1. Stand with your feet shoulder-width apart, and place your hands flat on the floor.

2. Walk your hands forward slowly, with your legs becoming as straight as possible at the knees, until you arrive in the downward-dog position. The vertical position of your arms will depend on your flexibility. If you are more flexible in your thighs and shoulders then your arms can be more vertical, and if you are less flexible your arms will be less vertical.

3. Begin to bend your elbows and lower yourself to the floor, balancing on your toes or flat feet if able. Try to keep your legs straight. If you are concerned about your head hitting the floor then have a cushion of some kind positioned under your head.

4. Continue bending your elbows until your face nearly touches the floor or until your elbows reach 90 degrees of bend.

5. Pause for a second, and then push back up to the starting position. This counts as one repetition.

Teaching Points

This exercise requires a "head-down" position and therefore has more safety considerations than the other Standards. If you are unsure about your ability to control the descending phase then have a cushion under the head. Also ensure that your hands and feet and unlikely to slip away from you as this could strain the lower back or cause you to fall on your head / face.

When To Progress

Once you can perform 3 reps without stopping, with full range of motion at the elbows and with straight knees, then you will have mastered another of the Seven Standards of body weight exercise!

To help you master the inverted shoulder press we have gathered together a set of preparatory exercises that will help in developing the necessary strength and function. These exercises are presented in the following sections, starting with the hamstring stretch.

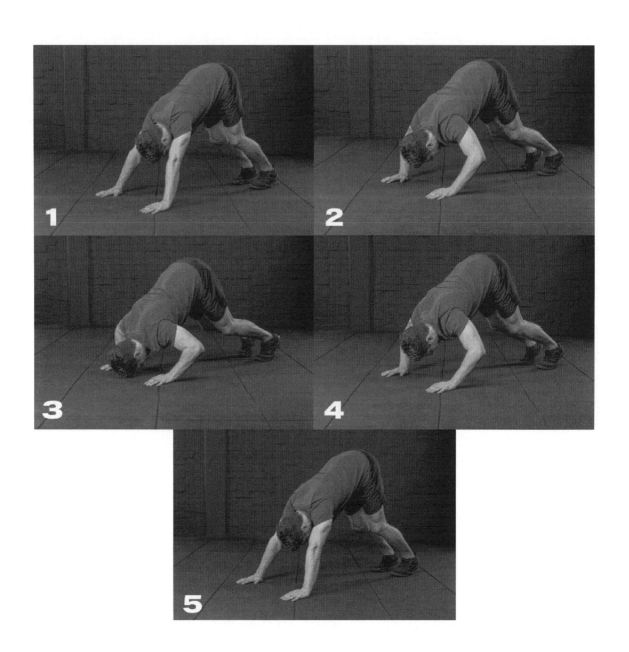

Hamstring Stretch

It may seem strange to include a hamstring stretch for what is essentially a shoulder strength exercise, but the inverted shoulder press requires a degree of hamstring flexibility and our experience has shown that many people have "tight" hamstrings. This exercise may also help with any tension and aches around the low back, hips and thighs.

Where To Do It

To perform the hamstring stretch you will need some floor space, and a mat if you need to cushion the ground. A carpeted floor may be adequate for comfort.

How To Do It

1. To perform the hamstring stretch, sit down on the floor with one leg out in front of you. Tuck your other leg into your buttocks and lay it flat on the floor.

2. Reach forward by bending at the hips, aiming to keep your back straight. You should feel the stretch in the back of the thigh in the straight leg. Focus on keeping the knee straight on the extended leg.

3. Move forwards until you feel a good stretch in the hamstrings. Hold for 20 seconds, change legs and repeat.

Teaching Points

The key to this exercise is to make sure that you are folding from the hips. If not, then you will get more of a back stretch than a hamstring stretch. Also, if you feel a pull in the back of the knee then bend it slightly. This will alleviate the strain but still allow you to stretch the hamstring. However if you bend the knee too much you will not be performing an effective stretch of the hamstring muscles at the back of the thigh.

When To Progress

Move onto the next stage when you can reach the toes on both feet with your hands, with a straight back, and bending from your hips. However, we recommend that you keep doing the hamstring stretch as part of your cool down, continuing to work on your hamstring flexibility to prevent any tightness and injury risk.

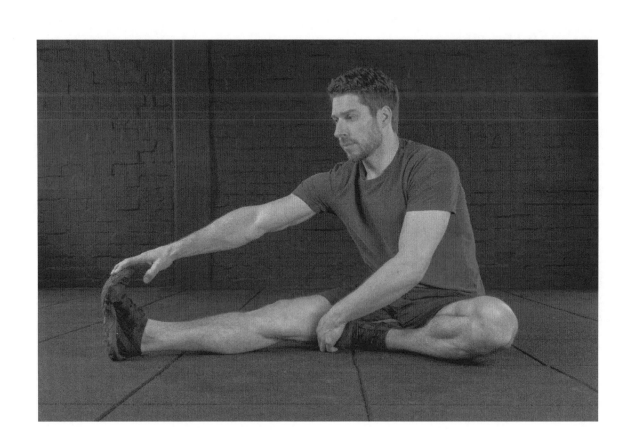

Bar Shoulder Stretch

As well as having tight hamstrings (see preparatory exercise 7.1), you may also have tight shoulders, and have limited motion around this joint. This is especially the case where you have a round-shouldered posture or have a history of heavy weight-lifting for the chest muscles. For this we recommend an accessible exercise to increase the flexibility of the shoulders. This is also a great exercise for creating a stretch through your middle-spine.

Where To Do It

You will need some space around and above you, and also a bar of some kind. Broom handles, exercise barbells, and anything long and straight will do the trick.

How To Do It

1. Stand with your feet slightly wider than shoulder width apart, and grab the bar with an overhand grip, hands as wide as you can comfortably get them. Make sure your elbows are not bent.

2. Begin with the bar resting in front of you, against your waist or tops of thighs. Now start to lift the bar up in a large arc, making sure to keep your arms straight.

3. Keep going until the bar is above and behind your head if possible. Hold this position for a few seconds as you feel the stretch, and then lower the bar and rest.

Teaching Points

If you have tight shoulders then you may struggle to keep your arms straight as the bar goes over your head. If this is the case then widen your grip on the bar. If the exercise is too easy, or you don't feel much of a stretch, then hold the bar with a closer grip.

When To Progress

Move on to the next stage when you can raise your arms above your head without feeling a stretch at the shoulders. It should be easy to get your arms above your head with a grip at shoulder width, and without undue stress at the chest or shoulders.

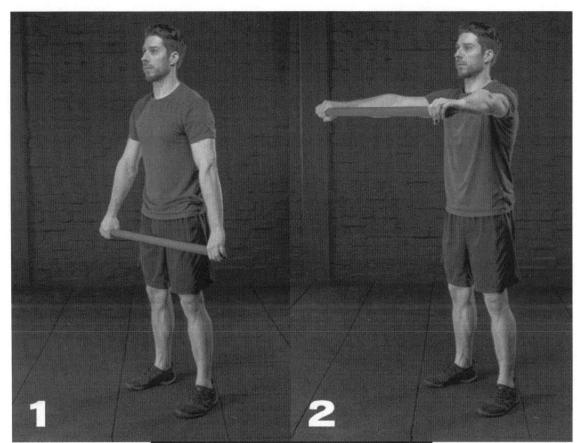

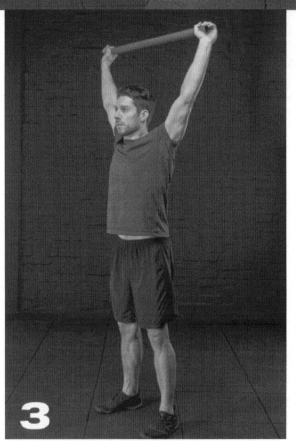

Downward Dog

We now come to an exercise that is popular in yoga: the downward dog. The downward dog is included here to increase your hamstring, shoulder, and middle-spine flexibility. It is therefore a combination of preparatory exercises 7.1 and 7.2. One further advantage to this exercise is that it will also develop strength in your upper body and trunk due to the static hold of body weight through the arms.

Where To Do It

To perform the downward dog you will need some floor space. Feel free to use a mat to stop your hands and feet from slipping on the ground.

How To Do It

1. Stand with your feet shoulder width apart, and then bend forward at the waist and place your hands flat on the floor.

2. Now start walking your hands forward slowly, one at a time, whilst keeping your knees as straight as possible and aiming to keep your heels down and in contact with the ground.

3. You should feel a strong stretch in the back of your legs. If you need to, bend your knees slightly to alleviate the stretch. You will also feel the strain of your body weight through your shoulders. Distribute this load through the middle of each hand as it contacts the ground.

4. Aim to hold the pose for 10 to 20 seconds initially. Focus on keeping a straight spine, elbows and knees.

Teaching Points

The main focus of the downward dog is to develop flexibility of your hamstrings, shoulders, and spine, so keep this in mind when doing the exercise. Try thinking about folding from the hips, and keeping a slight bend in the knee if needed. Distribute your body weight through the hands and feet, with your buttocks forming the highest point of your body.

When To Progress

You should progress when you can hold the downward dog for 30 seconds, with a 90-degree bend in your hips, straight knees, and heels in contact with the ground.

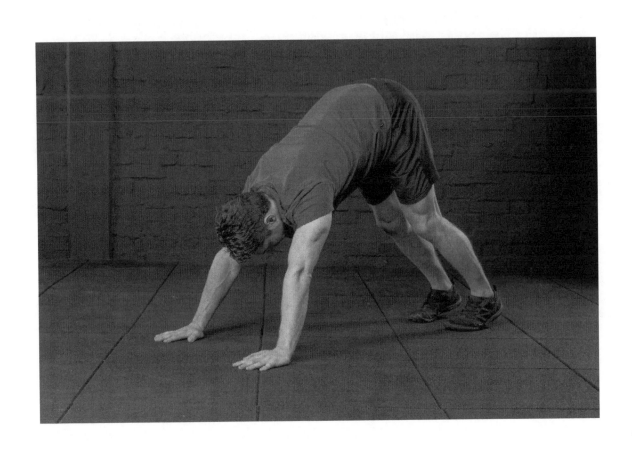

Kneeling Inverted Hold

The kneeling inverted hold is another static exercise, which means that there is no movement, but that the muscles are still working hard to hold your position against gravity. It is great for building muscle strength and stability in the shoulders! Please note, you should not do this exercise if you have a history of high blood pressure, gastric reflux, or any other condition that you are not sure about. If in doubt we recommend that you seek advice from a suitably qualified health or medical professional.

Where To Do It

You will need a platform to place your knees upon, and a floor with a non slip surface. For the platform you can use a chair, exercise step, or other solid object; as long as it is comfortable for your knees, and sturdy and will not move when you are on it.

How To Do It

1. Kneel down on the platform that you are using, resting your weight on your shins.

2. Grab the edge of the platform and slowly and carefully move your hands from the platform to the floor.

3. Position your hands on the floor with palms flat, shoulder width apart. Distribute the weight of your upper-body through the centre of your hands and through the middle finger. Keep the elbows straight.

4. Now lift your hips up so that your bum comes away from your shins. Keep going until you feel weight being moved onto your arms and shoulders. Stop when you feel enough resistance.

5. Keep your elbows straight throughout! Hold this position for as long as you can, initially 10 to 20 seconds. Then push yourself steadily back to the start position.

Teaching Points

Like the other preparatory exercises in this book that have a kneeling or platform component, exercise 7.4 can be adjusted with height to make it easier or more difficult. Use a lower platform to ease the exercise as this places less body weight onto the arms. As you get stronger and more confident you can move to a higher platform.

When To Progress

Move on to the next stage when you can hold the position for 30 seconds without resting, with your elbows straight and the arms approaching a vertical position.

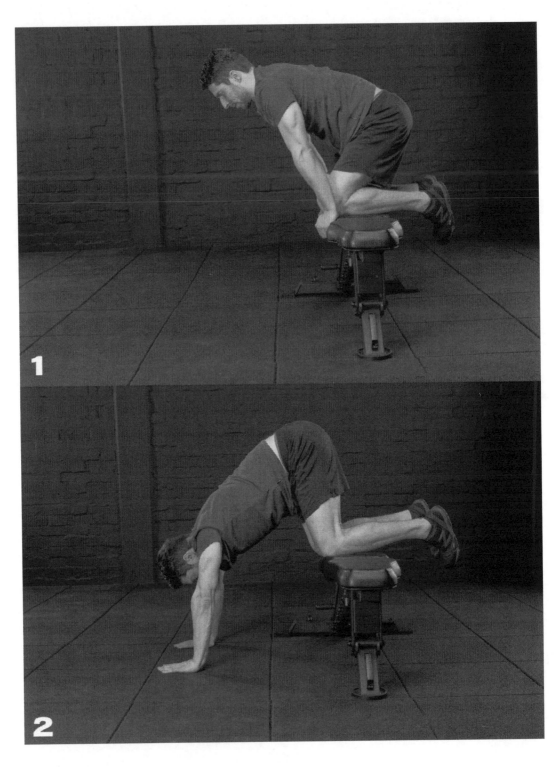

Kneeling Shallow Press

Building on the difficulty of preparatory exercise 7.4, we now come to the kneeling shallow press. If you have reached this stage then you are making great progress, as exercise 7.5 will allow you to get a good feeling for Standard Seven: The Inverted Shoulder Press, but from the safety of the knees. It will require a degree of shoulder strength and stability but will allow you to control the depth of the movement.

Please note, you should not do this exercise if you have a history of high blood pressure, gastric reflux, or any other condition that you are not sure about. If in doubt we recommend that you seek advice from a suitably qualified health or medical professional.

Where To Do It

You will need a platform to place your knees upon, and a floor with a non slip surface. For the platform you can use a chair, exercise step, or other solid object; as long as it is comfortable for your knees, and sturdy and will not move when you are on it.

How To Do It

1. Kneel down on the platform that you are using, resting your weight on your shins.

2. Grab the edge of the platform and slowly and carefully move your hands from the platform to the floor. Position your hands with palms flat, shoulder width apart.

3. Move forward until your arms are in a nearly vertical position, or as vertical as your flexibility, strength, and ability allows. Distribute the weight of your upper-body through the centre of your hands.

4. Bend your elbows and lower your head towards the floor. Be careful here, and only bend your elbows a small amount to start with (that is why this is called the shallow press). We recommend you place a cushion or similar under your head if you are new to this exercise and unsure as to whether or not you can support yourself on bent elbows.

5. At the end position, pause for a second, and then push back up to the start position by straightening the elbows. This counts as one repetition.

Teaching Points

Like the other preparatory exercises in this book that have a kneeling or platform component, exercise 7.5 can be adjusted with height to make it easier or more difficult. Use a lower platform to ease the exercise as this places less body weight onto the arms. As you get stronger and more confident you can move to a higher platform.

When To Progress

Move on to the next stage when you can do 5 reps with your elbows reaching at least 45 degrees of bend.

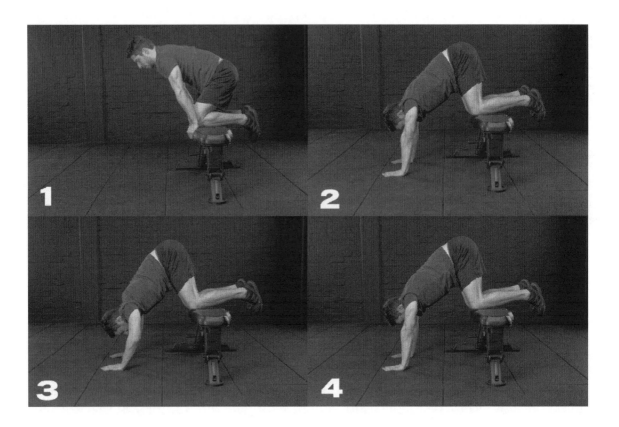

Full Kneeling Press

The full kneeling press is very similar to exercise 7.5, except that this time you should be trying to get your head as close to the ground as possible, or the elbows to bend at least 90 degrees, whichever occurs sooner. Be warned, this is a difficult exercise and requires good strength in the shoulders and arms. This increased resistance and greater depth of movement will build your upper body and core strength though, preparing you for the final stage - Standard Seven: The Inverted Shoulder Press!

Please note, you should not do this exercise if you have a history of high blood pressure, gastric reflux, or any other condition that you are not sure about. If in doubt we recommend that you seek advice from a suitably qualified health or medical professional.

Where To Do It

You will need a platform to place your knees upon, and a floor with a non slip surface. For the platform you can use a chair, exercise step, or other solid object; as long as it is comfortable for your knees, and sturdy and will not move when you are on it.

How To Do It

1. Kneel down on the platform that you are using, resting your weight on your shins.

2. Grab the edge of the platform and slowly and carefully move your hands from the platform to the floor. Position your hands with palms flat, shoulder width apart. Distribute your weight through the centre of your hands.

3. Move forward until your arms are in a nearly vertical position, or as vertical as your flexibility, strength, and ability allows.

4. Bend your elbows and lower yourself towards the floor. The aim is to get either your elbows at 90 degrees, or your head nearly touching the floor, whichever occurs sooner. You may opt to place a cushion or similar underneath your head for reassurance and safety.

5. At the bottom of the movement pause for a second, and then push back up to the start position by straightening your elbows. This counts as one repetition.

Teaching Points

The full kneeling press can be adjusted like preparatory exercises 7.4 and 7.5, by changing the height of the kneeling platform. A lower platform will make the exercise easier. The resistance of exercise 7.6 can also be modified by reducing the range of motion at the elbows.

When To Progress

Move on to the next stage when you can perform 5 reps without resting and without undue stress in the shoulders and arms.

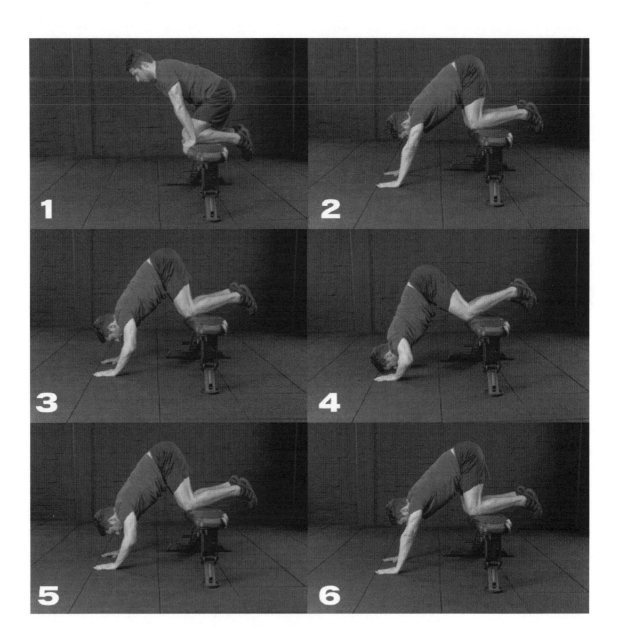

11. Programs

Knowing how to perform the exercises is one thing, but to make good progress you need structured exercise programs to keep you motivated. Structured exercise programs guide you through each workout, telling you how many reps to perform, how many sets to do, and how much rest time to take. The combination of exercise will vary to give a physically well-rounded routine that remains mentally interesting.

In this book we have 7 programs, each containing 7 exercises. They are:

- Preparatory Program 1
- Preparatory Program 2
- Preparatory Program 3
- Preparatory Program 4
- Preparatory Program 5
- Preparatory Program 6
- The Seven Standards Program

The exercises are structured in each program based on their relative potential difficulty. If you are completely new to exercise or body weight exercise then start with program 1. In any case we recommend you start at program 1, and if you find the exercises manageable then you get an immediate sense of achievement and you will ensure you have the required physical attributes for the next level program.

Lastly, we have structured and displayed our programs in a way that is as easy as possible to follow. Start at the top, and work your way down, following each instruction sequentially.

Adjusting the Programs

Although we have carefully considered each exercise and program to allow for the widest range of abilities, the huge variation between people means that these programs can only ever be a rough guide. Please refer back to each exercise description individually for teaching points on how to adapt the exercise to your ability level.

You can also adjust the rest time taken between each set. Reducing the rest time will make the programs harder, as your body will have less time to recover between each bout of exercise. Conversely, increasing the rest time between each set will make the programs easier, as your body will have more time to recover between each exercise.

Adjusting the number of reps will also adjust the difficulty. If you are struggling to perform the suggested number of reps then reduce them a little and see how you get on. Conversely, if you have reached the required number of reps, but do not feel ready to move on to the next program, increase the number of reps in each set to increase the challenge.

One last way of adjusting the programs is to adjust the number of sets. Decreasing the number of sets will make the programs easier, whilst increasing the number of sets will make the programs more difficult. It is recommended to decrease or increase the number of sets by the same amount across the board; that way you will not get confused as you move between exercises within the same program.

If you are still unsure of how to progress or adjust the programs to suit your particular ability level, then please get in touch. We can be reached via email at: **bodyweightbasics@mail.com**

11.1 Preparatory Program 1

Time required: 45 minutes to 1 hour
Frequency per week: 3 to 5, depending on your goals

If you are a complete beginner, are injured, or have not exercised for a long time, then this program is for you! First, do your warm up and stretch. Then, move onto the first exercise. Here you will perform the required number of reps, for the required number of sets, and take the required amount of rest time. Then move onto the second exercise and do the same, and then the third exercise, and then the fourth exercise, and so on. Lastly, you will do the cool down and stretch.

Preparatory Program 1	
Warm-up and stretch	
1	Kneeling Platform Push-up Perform 8 reps, then rest for 30 to 60 seconds. Repeat 3 times.
2	Standing Row Perform 3 reps, then rest for 30 to 60 seconds. Repeat 3 times.
3	Ledge Dip Knees Bent Perform 8 reps, then rest for 30 to 60 seconds. Repeat 3 times.
4	Kneeling Platform Push-up Perform 8 reps, then rest for 30 to 60 seconds. Repeat 3 times.
5	Sit Stand Perform 8 reps, then rest for 30 to 60 seconds. Repeat 3 times.
6	Prone Pelvic Tilt Perform 8 reps, then rest for 30 to 60 seconds. Repeat 3 times.
7	Hamstring Stretch Hold for 20 seconds on both legs
Cool down and stretch	
Finish	

11.2 Preparatory Program 2

Time required: 45 minutes to 1 hour
Frequency per week: 3 to 5, depending on your goals

Once you have developed some initial strength and mobility, you can start this routine, which is Preparatory Program 2. This is where you will start performing exercises that are very similar in nature to the Standards, except they are more accessible.

Preparatory Program 2	
Warm-up and stretch	
1	Kneeling Push-up Perform 8 reps, then rest for 30 to 60 seconds. Repeat 3 times.
2	Supine Row Perform 3 reps, then rest for 30 to 60 seconds. Repeat 3 times.
3	Ledge Dip With Straight Legs Perform 10 reps, then rest for 30 to 60 seconds. Repeat 3 times.
4	Shallow Squat Perform 10 reps, then rest for 30 to 60 seconds. Repeat 3 times.
5	Hip Flexor Stretch Hold for 30 seconds on each leg
6	Platform Push-up Hold Perform 15 seconds, then rest for 30 to 60 seconds. Repeat 3 times.
7	Bar Shoulder Stretch Perform 20 reps
Cool down and stretch	
Finish	

11.3 Preparatory Program 3

Time required: 45 minutes to 1 hour
Frequency per week: 3 to 5, depending on your goals

Now we're getting there! Preparatory Program 3 is where you start to progress onto more demanding variations of the Seven Standards. Be sure to follow the suggested sequences.

Preparatory Program 3	
Warm-up and stretch	
1	Platform Push-up Perform 8 reps, then rest for 30 to 60 seconds. Repeat 3 times.
2	Dead Hang Hold for 15 seconds, then rest for 30 to 60 seconds. Repeat 3 times.
3	Kneeling Triceps Push-up Perform 8 reps, then rest for 30 to 60 seconds. Repeat 3 times.
4	Shallow One Leg Squat Perform 5 reps on each leg, rest for 30 to 60 seconds. Repeat 3 times.
5	Lateral Lunge Perform 8 reps each way, then rest for 30 to 60 seconds. Repeat 3 times.
6	Bridge Hold for 15 seconds, then rest for 30 to 60 seconds. Repeat 3 times.
7	Downward Dog Hold for 20 seconds, then rest for 30 to 60 seconds. Repeat 2 times.
Cool down and stretch	
Finish	

11.4 Preparatory Program 4

Time required: 45 minutes to 1 hour
Frequency per week: 3 to 5, depending on your goals

We're really progressing now! Preparatory Program 4 is where real strength is built. Negative versions of the push-up, as well as shallow triceps dips are included here, to start testing your ability.

Preparatory Program 4	
Warm-up and stretch	
1	Negative Push-up Perform 1 rep for 15 seconds, rest for 30 to 60 seconds. Repeat 3 times.
2	Pull-up Pulses Perform 5 reps, then rest for 30 to 60 seconds. Repeat 3 times.
3	Shallow Triceps Dip Perform 5 reps, then rest for 30 to 60 seconds. Repeat 3 times.
4	Crouch Hold for 15 seconds, then rest for 30 to 60 seconds. Repeat 3 times.
5	Shallow Lunge Perform 8 reps on each leg, rest for 30 to 60 seconds. Repeat 3 times.
6	Kneeling Plank Hold for 15 seconds, then rest for 30 to 60 seconds. Repeat 3 times.
7	Kneeling Inverted Hold Hold for 15 seconds, then rest for 30 to 60 seconds. Repeat 3 times.
Cool down and stretch	
Finish	

11.5 Preparatory Program 5

Time required: 45 minutes to 1 hour
Frequency per week: 3 to 5, depending on your goals

Moving on we now arrive at Preparatory Program 5. We are nearing the goal exercises now, and so this stage has many negative versions and slightly easier variations of the Standard exercises. This means that your strength should be building at a steady rate now, and you should see some progress every week.

	Preparatory Program 5
	Warm-up and stretch
1	Static Hold Push-up Hold for 30 seconds, then rest for 30 to 60 seconds. Repeat 3 times.
2	Negative Pull-up Perform 1 rep for 15 seconds, rest for 30 to 60 seconds. Repeat 3 times.
3	Negative Triceps Dip Perform 1 rep for 15 seconds, rest for 30 to 60 seconds. Repeat 3 times.
4	Assisted Squat Perform 8 reps, then rest for 30 to 60 seconds. Repeat 3 times.
5	Lunge Balance Perform 8 reps, then rest for 30 to 60 seconds. Repeat 3 times.
6	Static Crunch Hold for 15 seconds, then rest for 30 to 60 seconds. Repeat 3 times.
7	Kneeling Shallow Press Perform 3 reps, then rest for 30 to 60 seconds. Repeat 3 times.
	Cool down and stretch
	Finish

11.6 Preparatory Program 6

Time required: 45 minutes to 1 hour
Frequency per week: 3 to 5, depending on your goals

Preparatory Program 6 is the last program before you tackle the ultimate program containing the Seven Standards! Many of these exercises may take an extended period of time to adapt to so don't be surprised if you spend weeks or even months on this stage. Don't rush your progress, you will be building strength and your physical ability all the time!

Preparatory Program 6	
Warm-up and stretch	
1	Shallow Push-up Perform 8 reps, then rest for 30 to 60 seconds. Repeat 3 times.
2	Assisted Pull-up Perform 5 reps, then rest for 30 to 60 seconds. Repeat 3 times.
3	Assisted Triceps Dip Perform 5 reps, then rest for 30 to 60 seconds. Repeat 3 times.
4	Deep Squat Position Hold for 20 seconds, then rest for 30 to 60 seconds. Repeat 3 times.
5	Static Lunge Perform 8 reps on each leg, rest for 30 to 60 seconds. Repeat 3 times.
6	Plank Pulses Perform 8 reps, then rest for 30 to 60 seconds. Repeat 3 times.
7	Full Kneeling Press Perform 3 reps, then rest for 30 to 60 seconds. Repeat 3 times.
Cool down and stretch	
Finish	

11.7 The Seven Standards Program

Time required: 45 minutes to 1 hour
Frequency per week: 3 to 5, depending on your goals

You're nearly there! This program is the real deal, the Seven Standards Program. In this you will work with all seven of the goal exercises, training to achieve the goal number of reps. You will follow the guided number of sets and reps, trying to complete the program in a single workout session.

You will see for example that the push-up is listed as 3 sets of 8 reps. The goal is to be able to do 8 reps of the push-up without stopping, and so performing 3 sets of 5 reps is the best way to build this strength in a progressive way. Every week or two it is best to test yourself and see if you can hit the goal number of reps. If you can, well done, you have mastered another Standard exercise! If not, keep training and try again in two weeks. Eventually you will meet the rep requirement and master all Seven Standards!

Seven Standards Program	
Warm-up and stretch	
1	Push-up Perform 8 reps, then rest for 30 to 60 seconds. Repeat 3 times.
2	Pull-up Perform 3 reps, then rest for 30 to 60 seconds. Repeat 3 times.
3	Triceps Dip Perform 8 reps, then rest for 30 to 60 seconds. Repeat 3 times.
4	Squat Perform 8 reps, then rest for 30 to 60 seconds. Repeat 3 times.
5	Lunge Perform 8 reps, then rest for 30 to 60 seconds. Repeat 3 times.
6	Plank Perform 8 reps, then rest for 30 to 60 seconds. Repeat 3 times.
7	Inverted Shoulder Press Perform 3 reps, then rest for 30 to 60 seconds. Repeat 3 times.
Cool down and stretch	
Finish	

11.8 Where To Go Next

Once you have mastered the Seven Standards you might be wondering where you should go next in your fitness journey. There are many routes that you can take once you have built the basic level of strength with our Seven Standard exercises.

One route to take is to simply keep doing the Seven Standards, and slight variations of these, for the rest of the time that you exercise. Your physical strength will be more than adequate for almost anything you face in everyday life. You don't even have to add more reps or sets, as effectively this will be a maintenance program.

If you wish to start doing weights and move on to more advanced forms of exercise then mastering the Seven Standards will be a very good base to launch from. You will find that the transition from body weight exercise to weighted exercise much easier if you have this base level of strength and fitness. Your joints, soft tissues and muscles will be well prepared for the new loads.

If you wish to continue your body weight training, but at a more advanced level, then you can check out *Complete Calisthenics - The Ultimate Guide To Body weight Exercise*, by Ashley Kalym. This book starts where *Body Weight Basics* finishes, and builds on the Seven Standards with many new and challenging exercises. *Complete Calisthenics* will take you to new heights and will show you ways in which you can advance the exercises you already know, such as the push-up and pull-up.

12. Frequently Asked Questions

As you're likely new to exercise, and resistance exercise specifically, you probably have loads of questions that might not have been answered so far. In this last section we are going to go through some of the most common questions that people have about resistance training and body weight training. If your question isn't answered here, then get in touch by email, and we'll do out best to help you! We can be reached at: bodyweightbasics@mail.com

Q. I've never exercised. Is it too late for me? Can I still do the exercises in this book?

A. It is never too late! Any physical activity will have a beneficial impact on your health, wellbeing, and physical ability, and as they say - "better late than never!" The exercises in this book are specifically designed for people that have not exercised before, are completely new to body weight training, or have a history of injury or immobility. In addition, we start each standard with the easiest possible variation, and give information on how to progress steadily through each stage, until you can master the Seven Standards we have chosen.

Q. My friend says that I am wasting my time with body weight exercise. Wouldn't I be better off using weights instead?

A. Not at all! Although exercising with free-weights or resistance machines gives great benefits, we think that if you cannot do the essential body weight exercises then your body lacks fundamental strength, mobility and control. Body weight exercise teaches body awareness, muscular control, balance, and the mobility of your joints. Working with free-weights and resistance machines can also do this, but in many cases large parts of the body are immobilised and so you may not develop the physical attributes mentioned above, especially for beginners who do already have these abilities. Also, perfecting body weight movements makes transitioning to using free-weights or resistance machines much more straightforward, as can be seen by the success of gymnasts.

Q. Is it necessary to join a gym?

A. No, we wouldn't say that it is necessary, although there are benefits to both exercising from home and at a gym. Exercising from home has obvious benefits; you don't have to travel in order to workout, you will feel comfortable and not self conscious, and the very nature of body weight exercise means that little to no equipment is needed for the vast majority of the exercises. The downsides to exercising at home are that you may struggle to get motivated to workout, exercising on your own might become a little lonely at times, and some pieces of equipment (like the assisted pull-up and triceps dip machine) you are unlikely to have, and are unlikely to buy (as they are expensive).

The benefits to joining a gym are that it is perfectly set -up for exercise and working out. It will have every piece of equipment that is needed for the exercises in this book (in the few exercises that require equipment), and there will be people there that can help or answer any questions that we have not covered here. The downsides to exercising in a gym are that it can be busy at certain times of the day, you will have to travel to your workout location, and the gym environment may be an uncomfortable environment for you. With body weight exercise, in the vast majority of exercises, you can exercise anytime, anywhere, including outdoors!

At the end of the day we think that belonging to a gym is a positive thing, and we have had only good experiences when exercising in such environments, but they can become monotonous after a while.

Q. Once I can do the Seven Standards, where do I go from there?

A. We're glad you asked! In all honesty, there are so many different types of training that it really is up to you.

In terms of body weight exercise there are hundreds of different exercises, and just as many variations available out there. Ashley has previously written a book looking at body weight training in more depth, called *Complete Calisthenics - The Ultimate Guide To body weight Exercise*. This book picks up where Body weight Basics finishes, and looks at more advanced movements such as the muscle-up, handstand, planche, back lever, L-sit, single leg squat, and many more.

You may also decide to progress onto weighted exercise, with dumbbells, barbells, and other forms of resistance training. The grounding that you get from mastering the seven standards will stand you in good stead for this journey as well, and help you to get to grips with the new type of exercise much faster than if you could not do the Seven Standards of Body weight Basics.

Q. Once I have mastered the Seven Standards, do I need to keep moving forwards?

A. No, you don't! Mastering the Seven Standards will take some time, depending on your starting ability. But, even if you got to the target level suggested in this book, and then never went any further, this would still allow you to enjoy a level of strength and physical ability that many people lack.

Obviously, to keep the level of fitness that you achieve you will have to keep training. As the saying goes, "if you don't use it, you lose it". You will find that maintenance of your fitness levels is far easier than getting there in the first place. Also, you will find that the ability to perform the Seven Standards will give you more than enough strength, agility, and physical robustness for nearly every daily physical task that life throws at you.

Q. I'm prone to a few injuries, should I still do body weight exercise?

A. Absolutely! The authors (that's Ross and Ashley, again) have previously written a book specifically demonstrating how body weight exercise can be used both to prevent and rehabilitate musculoskeletal injuries. *Bulletproof Bodies: Body Weight Exercise for Injury Prevention and Rehabilitation* uses a range of body weight strength and mobility exercises not seen in *Body Weight Basics*, and tailors these to a range of common musculoskeletal injuries seen in various joints and soft tissues. *Bulletproof Bodies* will also teach you some background to each injury so that you can better understand your physical limitations and potential. These exercises can supplement any advice you have received from a Physiotherapist or medical doctor.

Printed in Great Britain
by Amazon

31849959R00093